HOW TO BUILD A BODY THAT LASTS

Adam Richardson is the UK's top trending health and fitness coach with a rapidly growing audience across both TikTok and Instagram. Adam is passionate about removing barriers to exercise and movement, a philosophy that is key to his work as a personal trainer in which he strives to help his clients feel more confident, as well as more fit and healthy.

HOW TO BUILD A BODY THAT LASTS

Exercises for Longevity, Strength and Health

ADAM RICHARDSON

CENTURY

1 3 5 7 9 10 8 6 4 2

Century
20 Vauxhall Bridge Road
London SW1V 2SA

Century is part of the Penguin Random House group of companies whose
addresses can be found at global.penguinrandomhouse.com

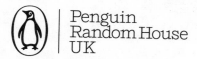

Penguin
Random House
UK

First published by Century in 2024

www.penguin.co.uk

A CIP catalogue record for this book is available from the British Library.

ISBN: 9781529928617

Illustrations by Richard Palmer

Typeset in 11.7/16 pt Calluna by Jouve (UK), Milton Keynes
Printed and bound in Great Britain by Clays Ltd, Elcograf S.p.A.

The authorised representative in the EEA is Penguin Random House Ireland,
Morrison Chambers, 32 Nassau Street, Dublin D02 YH68

www.greenpenguin.co.uk

Penguin Random House is committed to a sustainable future
for our business, our readers and our planet. This book is made
from Forest Stewardship Council® certified paper.

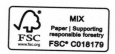

To Mar, Tara & Gwen.
I hope this body lasts, so we can enjoy this life together
for as long as possible!

Contents

Welcome to The Wiggle Room!

Hello, you ray of sunshine! First of all, I want to thank you for buying this book. Secondly, I want *you* to thank you for buying this book. I'm usually sceptical of any product or person that makes life-changing claims, but I genuinely believe the information in this book *will* change your life for the better, the way it has mine. I want to help you feel better, for longer. The secret to building a body that lasts? Mobility. Mobility is the foundation of a thriving existence, and that's exactly what we're here to do – make your life better, one wiggle at a time.

This is a fitness book – sort of. It's a book that will help you become fitter and healthier, but hopefully it won't feel like *just* a fitness book. Instead, I wanted to write a book about *you*; about how to get the most out of your life by teaching you how to extract the very best from your body for as long as possible without having to do anything too extreme.

I want to show you a different side to fitness. One that celebrates how you feel rather than just how you look, and hopefully doesn't feel too daunting. You'll learn all about that suit of meat and bones that carries you everywhere and what makes it so special, and pick up numerous tips and tricks to keep it running smoothly in the long run. Consider this my 'realistic approach to fitness for people who want to live in a body that feels good but don't really know where to start'. Very soon you'll understand what this mobility malarkey is all about and find what matters most to you as a unique individual with hopes, dreams and desires. We'll work through 20 exercises that will challenge your body in the best possible way, and explore all the weird and wonderful ways your body parts can (and can't yet) move. I'll be coaching you through my go-to mobility manoeuvres that need nothing more than a body, some mild enthusiasm and occasionally the odd thing lying around your house. Plus, I'll shower you with all my mobility moulding golden nuggets of how to actually make this movement habit stick, by finding ways to get more wiggle into your life.

Reaching a point where I actually enjoy fitness didn't happen overnight. There was a long period where I was just too embarrassed to step foot in the gym on my own, and the last thing I wanted to do was work out. But I have finally figured out what it was I was looking for, and I want to share with you the discoveries I've made through building my own movement habit. I believe it is something that everyone can benefit from, and that it can be truly transformative. But you know what they say – you have to be in it to win it.

We all have a different relationship with exercise. We know it is good for us – that's not exactly breaking news. Some people have a natural affinity for it and depend on fitness activities to get through their day. For others, the whole culture of exercise feels totally alien. I started exercising for the same reason that most people do: *because I wanted to be sexier.* If I'm honest, I wanted to stop looking like a pencil and I thought that growing some muscle and having abs would help me feel a little more confident in my own skin. What I didn't anticipate was that the constant focus on how I looked would start to suck the life out of my soul and only leave me feeling emptier.

I had spent most of my early twenties living in a body that felt about 70 years old. I couldn't help but think 'this isn't normal'. My back hurt, my hips and knees ached, and my shoulders liked to dislocate whenever they wanted. It felt like a constant battle against injury and stiffness, alongside this empty obsession with how much fat I had on my stomach. In a weird way, exercising ended up having a negative impact on my overall wellbeing, but it wasn't the moving that was doing the damage, it was how I perceived and used exercise that was the problem. I think deep down we all know that exercise is one of the single most impactful things that any of us can do for our physical and mental wellbeing, but like all good things, there is such a thing as too much.

Although my desire to look like Brad Pitt in *Fight Club* got me exercising in the first place, over time my priorities started to shift away from the mirror. For me, it had stopped being a positive because of *how* I was exercising. I was beating myself up, mentally and physically, and wondering why I didn't feel very good. Cutting a very long-winded story short, I had an epiphany; one that subsequently inspired a large proportion of my career trajectory and this book: one day, if I'm lucky, I'm going to resemble an old soggy tea bag, and how I look won't really matter. But how I feel *will*. My boobs may be sagging, and my biceps likely lagging, but if my body still works, hopefully I'll still be shagging. I wanted my body to stop hurting and for it to stay not hurting for as long as possible, which is what drove me down the mobility lane. I've never looked back, and that is what brings me to where we are today.

To be clear, I don't believe there's anything wrong with wanting to look a little better in your body. Who doesn't want to be sexier? I still train for aesthetic reasons, and I'd be lying if I said otherwise. But my purpose has shifted away from purely how I look to how I *feel* as well, and *mamma mia*, do I feel more fulfilled because of it. These musings about my experiences with exercise may feel like I'm plucking the thoughts from your brain – perhaps you too have these same feelings of dissatisfaction with your body. Regardless of your personal relationship with exercise, one thing I'm confident of is that if you choose to take on the information in this book, you'll feel more fulfilled. This book offers a blueprint to an improved relationship with your body, helping you move better than ever before, and hopefully discover a whole new perspective on how to make exercise work for you along the way.

The feeling of discomfort in my own skin is what got me going in the first place, and I'm grateful for the younger me, even though he had no idea what he was doing. I'm grateful he started this ball rolling because I wouldn't be here otherwise. So if, like me, you've reached a point where you're tired of striving to achieve an unrealistic standard pushed by society, feel underwhelmed by a body that keeps letting you down, and fatigued by exercise which feels like punishment, you've come to the right place. If you want to develop habits that make you feel *good*, habits that support and nurture gratitude towards the only body you'll ever live in, and find a way to enjoy doing the things you love, now and for a long, long time, then I'm excited for you to see what I have in store for you. Welcome to *How to Build a Body That Lasts.*

Love,
Adam xxx

What is Mobility?

So, what is this mobility malarkey that is the secret to longevity? Simply put, mobility is 'the ability to move freely and easily'. Aka your movement ability ('mo-bility' – get it?). In other words, the not-so-sexy yet fundamental aspect of health and fitness that I believe is key to squeezing as much juice as possible out of this short life of ours. There are countless benefits to improving your mobility. The overarching purpose of mobility training is movement freedom – developing the ability to move the way you need to, in order to do the things you want to do and live an independent life. But what are the specific benefits to training your mobility?

If you incorporate mobility training into your life, you will:

- Develop stronger, more robust joints and muscles, which are able to more readily cope with the stresses of life and activities of your choice.
- Improve your flexibility and become more supple, helping you to move through daily life with greater ease.
- Reduce joint stiffness and pain by building happier and healthier joints.
- Better your balance, reducing the risk of falls.
- Reduce risk of injury by regularly exposing and readying your body for what the world is going to throw at you.
- Increase longevity and quality of life by helping you to stay active, now and in the future.

- Improve your relationship with your body through greater bodily awareness.
- Reduce stress and improve energy and mood.

This isn't an exhaustive list, and there are countless benefits beyond the more obvious physical ones listed here that you'll discover as you wiggle through the rest of this book.

Perhaps it's even more powerful to imagine what your life would be like *without* full mobility. What would your time on this planet look like if you suddenly couldn't move freely and easily? What would your day-to-day life be like if the things you now find easy suddenly felt impossible? Maybe this is what you're facing right now. Maybe you're struggling with certain aspects of your mobility. Maybe you've been injured or live with a disability or chronic pain and know exactly how it feels to struggle through your day.

Or maybe you're one of the lucky ones, who – touch wood – has never *really* struggled to move but simply wants to feel better overall. While I'll never know your individual life circumstances and what makes you *you,* I'm confident that we can both agree, irrespective of where you are now, that life is really bloody tough when you can't move freely and easily. Mobility underpins almost everything we do and is one of the foundations of an independent life. Of course, mobility training isn't a magic pill that will rid you of any and every problem in your body. But if, like me, physical independence is important to you and you want to be clicking your heels, playing with your kids, your grandkids, your cat and your dog, and wiping your own bum for as long as possible, then it's probably a good idea to start paying into your 'movement pension' sooner rather than later.

For the most part, the body does a bloody good job at carrying us through, albeit with bumps along the road. I'm sure there are a fair few of you who have experienced the feeling that your body just isn't working the way you'd like it to. Whether it's pain in the knee, a sore back or a constant stiff feeling you can't seem to shake, these discomforts are something we'll all know at some point in our lives. But no matter how old or how stiff you might be, I don't believe it is ever too late to reap the rewards of mobility training. I can't remember where I heard it, but this proverb seems appropriate: 'the best time to plant a tree was twenty years ago, the next best time is now'. When you picked up this book, you planted the seed of your mobility, and with every page you read, you water and tend to that seed a little bit more.

Our ability to move is one of those beautiful things that seems so simple, until suddenly it doesn't. We spend years as little bambinos learning how to coordinate our rapidly growing body, falling flat on our bums and sometimes our faces hundreds of times a day – just to learn how to balance our big heads and stand on our own two feet. But by the time we're old enough to appreciate how much effort goes into learning to move, to walk, to talk, or even just use a spoon without making a mess, every aspect of our mobility almost feels like a given – like it's always been there. And like most of the good things in life, you don't know what you got 'til it's gone. Simple movements like climbing the stairs, walking, running, standing up, sitting down, or even just putting socks on – movements that we once glided through without so much as a second thought – can start to feel a little more clunky and painful, and paired with plenty of moans and groans, even at the not-so-ripe age of 30. It's hard not to sound preachy while passionately proclaiming 'it doesn't have to be this way', but I genuinely believe it doesn't. All we have to do is learn how to tend to our body by moving it the way it wants us to. That's what this method is all about: learning to listen to your body and give it what it truly needs.

Improving mobility isn't just about avoiding ailments as we hurtle past middle age and into our golden years. The last thing I want is to fill you with the fear that it's all downhill from here. I don't believe dread is the best motivator and, anyway, there's plenty of life to live *now*. This method is about valuing and making the most of what we have while we have it, as much as looking after our future selves. Although eventual physical decline is unavoidable, there are 70-year-olds busting out the splits, 80-year-olds deadlifting their bodyweight, and 90-year-olds running marathons, still living life to the full, fuelled by their ability to move. Equally, there's the 24-year-old version of me who's scared to sneeze in case he puts his back out again. While I don't believe for a second that anyone requires extreme mobility to thrive, the reality is that *your age is defined by your mobility; your mobility is not defined by your age.* If you're tired of feeling older than you are, it all starts with moving more now, regardless of where you're starting out.

I find myself thinking about my grandad, Ron, while writing this. (You don't meet babies called Ron these days, do you?) My grandad was always an active bean. Not in a sporty or athletic sense, though he was always mobile and had no problem chasing us around as young whippersnappers. Whether I was passing a ball around his garden or being bored to death walking around a train museum, I never once doubted his ability to move. But in the last of my grandad's 82 years, he found it impossible to walk more than 100 metres without having to stop because of excruciating pain in his legs. He was a stubbornly proud man and refused to walk with a cane, or much support at all, and sadly within a year he died. He was a sensational grandad, but towards the end, as he stopped stomping about and found himself chained to his chair, and his ability to move diminished, so did his lust for life. I'll never really know how my grandad felt at this point, but one thing I can say for certain is that the ability to move freely and easily, and the independence that comes with it, plays a monumental role in making life what it is.

If I'm one of the lucky ones that makes it to 80 before popping my clogs, I want to be able to look back, beaming with pride, saying, 'Cor, I gave that a bloody good go, I've had a great innings.' But I'm not going to wait until then to grasp what I have now, wishing I'd used my body while I had the chance. Instead, I'm going to do my bloody best to take care of it and value it for everything it does for me while I can. It can be really hard to feel thankful for our body at times, especially if it may not be quite working how you want it to. But you and I are going to strive to find a glimmer of gratitude over the following pages by learning more about *your body*, and discovering how to speak its language, so you can take care of it the way it needs. In other words, we're going to get our wiggle on, explore our bodies, and find simple ways of sprinkling movement into our lives that *finally* stick. I like to imagine I'm the 80-year-old version of me, looking back over my life. What would old man Adam be grateful for? What would he wish he could have a helping of in his older age? What do I have now that I don't even notice that would be life-enhancing for the future me?

Thankfully you're already reading this book, so your mobility ball is rolling, and as you'll discover throughout this movement manifesto, I don't believe you need to do anything wild and drastic to make the most of your body (unless you really want to). It's more about understanding your baseline, discovering the right amount for *you*, and working within your Goldilocks Zone. I'm going to encourage each of you to become your own scientist and explore how to make movement fit your life and your needs. What we're looking for is the not too much but not too little window (thus Goldilocks), finding just the right amount of movement to allow you to build a resilient body that keeps you on your feet for as long as possible.

Who Is It For?

The beauty of mobility training is that it really is for everyone. That might feel a little like a seedy sales line, but whether you're my 89-year-old nan or a bodybuilder, an avid gardener or a gym buff, mobility training is the one form of fitness that bridges age and lifestyle. If you want to move better, then mobility training is for you. It isn't just one style of training, however. Without sounding like I'm inviting you to join a cult, mobility is more of a concept than a specific training style and there's plenty of wiggle room in how you train to improve your mobility – hence the title of the introduction (punbelievable).

We will explore why movement is important to you as a unique human being, and how to build and maintain your general mobility. We'll test your movements with a series of challenges that also double up as incredible mobility exercises, and interpret what they tell us about how your body works and how we can make your day-to-day life easier by practising and refining your movement skills. Then we will discover how you can seamlessly integrate these moves into your life, and how to adopt a 'less is more' attitude to exercise to help stick with it, while providing you with a mobility training programme that you can adapt to your own level and time availability. On top of this, I'll be busting a few myths around health and fitness, revealing the nonsense you don't need to worry about, and hopefully making you smile along the way.

While it's impossible to create something for *everyone*, I've done my best to make *How to Build a Body That Lasts* as accessible and inclusive as I can, and I believe this approach is more than enough to help most of us live a wonderfully wiggle-filled life. If you choose to, you can use this movement foundation to work towards some fancier, more specific mobility goals. But for now, the aim of *How to Build a Body That Lasts* is to give you a well-rounded footing on which to build your movement hopes and dreams. I want to inspire you to see how incredible your body is and can be, and hopefully help you frolic into the later stages of your life. And all of this without having to step foot inside a gym.

BREATHE

Throughout this book I'm going to be throwing a lot of challenges at you, all of them aimed at improving your mobility.

For the first challenge, all I need you to do is to:

Take a really big, deep breath and breathe it all out.
Repeat this as many times as you like.

I'm not going to tell you how to breathe – after all, you've managed so far, haven't you? The only thing I'm going to ask is that you take a big, deep breath and sigh it out slowly. Nice and relaxed. Feels good, doesn't it?

Breathing is an amazing automatic function that our brain seems to have under control without us having to pay too much attention to it. Imagine how difficult life would be if we had to consciously coordinate that all day? But every now and again, it's a good idea to consciously control our breath and make sure our lungs, ribs and all the muscles in between are expanded to their full capacity. When was the last time you took a really deep breath? Not only does this work incredibly well at snapping us back to the present moment, but it also helps to steady our heart rate and relax our muscles.

If, like me, you find yourself unconsciously holding tension, maybe shrugging your shoulders to your ears or clenching your jaw without realising, taking a deep breath is a sensational way of physically and mentally resetting. This is your moment to hit that refresh button. We all know we should take regular breaks throughout the day, but the toughest part of that is remembering to do it. So, throughout this book I'm going to nudge you every now and again, and remind you to take a big, deep breath and chill your beans.

What does breathing have to do with mobility, I hear you ask? Not only is this breathing business important for keeping us alive, but it stops us from becoming too tense while we move. Being able to breathe calmly and in a controlled manner is a great sign that we're in control of an exercise. As we dive into the parts of the book that cover physical movement, we'll explore how to use the breath to improve mobility.

Every time you see the word BREATHE throughout this book, I want you to use it as a little prompt to dip out of the madness, bring yourself back to earth, fill those beautiful lungs with some delicious oxygen, and most importantly – *relax*.

So, for good measure, let's take one more big breath before we look at what mobility actually is.

Key Features of Mobility

It's safe to say that movement can get pretty bloody complicated, especially when we get into the detail of how your brain works with your body. As a result of our sensational supercomputer (our brain) and its ability to simplify complex calculations into easily digestible nuggets, it feels like movement just 'happens'. We're lucky we don't have to put much active thought into moving each individual muscle, joint and bone, otherwise life would be a logistical nightmare. However, this automation has a habit of leaving us in sticky situations if left on autopilot for too long. Our brain is constantly making what we subconsciously perceive as the most efficient and effective decisions when it comes to solving the problem of how we move. While this is great for preventing information overload, it can mean that we end up stuck in a movement rut, and our body defaults into using the same patterns again and again with little variety. And of course, if there's one thing our body needs, it's movement variety – which we all know is the spice of life.

We'll explore the brain's computing ability in more detail later in the book, but for now we're just going to marvel at our mysterious supercomputer and simplify our movement processes into a few key components to better understand how we can harness the benefits of mobility for our body. These key components are balance and coordination, strength, flexibility and endurance. Essentially, we're looking at our ability to move through a given range of motion. This requires control and coordination through movements, with enough flexibility and strength so that we don't crumble, snap and become knackered too quickly. Our job is to develop sufficient ability in all of these areas so that we can confidently do the things that are important to us without too much pain and difficulty along the way. Unfortunately for us humans, there's one unavoidable truth about movement: if you don't use it, you lose it.

Practice Makes Progress

The body has an incredible ability to adapt, but in order to stimulate adaptation, we have to expose ourselves to specific things, and here I introduce a fundamental principle of the human body: the SAID principle. This loud-looking acronym stands for 'Specific Adaptation to Imposed Demands', and as you might have guessed, it encompasses the ways in which the body adapts specifically in response to the demands and stresses placed on it. In layman's terms, if you want to get better at something, you have to practise it. If you want to get better at cooking, you must cook. If you want to get better at painting, you must paint, and if you want to get better at moving, you have to move. Therefore, to improve our mobility we must expose our body to things that challenge our balance, coordination, strength, flexibility and endurance, and train these elements by regularly and progressively exposing our body to physical challenges that stimulate and maintain adaptation, allowing us to move more freely.

Say you want to get better at improving a specific area of your mobility, like touching your toes: you would need to spend more time reaching towards your toes. If you want to get better at holding a squat, you need to spend more time in a squat (I'm sure you get the point). Of course there are other things we can and will do alongside targeted movement to support our mobility mission and progress faster, but fundamentally this specificity is essential, and the more we expose the body to these exact positions, over time it will adapt to allow us to perform them with greater ease.

This can be tricky when a particular activity, such as a squat or touching your toes, is simply too difficult or painful to even attempt. And if that's where you are, then telling you to *just do more of that thing* becomes a bit useless. This is where we need to regress the movement and find a simpler variation, which is challenging but not impossible, and work up from there. This is known as graded or gradual exposure, and it allows you to train for the specific task at hand without overwhelming you by asking too much of your body too soon. Graded exposure is a fundamental aspect of *How to Build a Body That Lasts* and something we'll talk about in much more detail later in the book, including my 5-step method to help you work around painful movements (page 277).

You may be wondering what makes mobility training different from any other form of fitness, such as strength or resistance training (basically fancy ways of saying lifting weights). There's a huge amount of crossover where strength training often leads to improvements in mobility, and mobility training often leads to improvements in strength; that's because mobility training is essentially low-impact resistance training. The main difference is where we shine the spotlight. Strength training focuses more on our muscles and less on what's happening at the joint. Yes, muscles are also a key focus in mobility training, but rather than just making them really beefy, what we're zooming in on is how well our joints work; on our ability to *stretch and control* the muscles and connective tissue surrounding the joints across their designed range of motion. In practice this means regularly exposing our joints and muscles to progressively increasing loads across greater ranges of motion over time. The aim of the game is to stimulate changes to the body which allow you to move with control over larger ranges of motion or improve control within ranges of motion you already have access to. In short, to become stronger, bendier and more supple and for the context of this book, we'll be doing that using little more than your own body.

Contrary to popular belief (I'm not sure why those words make me feel rather fancy, but they do), mobility training isn't *just* stretching. Although stretching will play an important role in mobilising our body, it's just one element of a rather large movement puzzle that we'll piece together throughout our movement montage.

How Much Do You Need to Do?

How much mobility you need will depend on what you want to be able to do. If you have minimal athletic desires and just want to be able to get up off the floor, you won't need the same level of mobility as a gymnast who needs to bust out the splits. That's why this method is all about identifying where you are now and building on your unique baseline towards your goal. To do that, you'll undertake a series of movement challenges to find your ground zero. You'll be looking to master simple exercises while also learning how to pick the 'lowest hanging fruit' when it comes to improving your mobility, in order to get the biggest bang for your buck for the least amount of input.

For a long time, I felt as though every workout had to leave me in a sweaty, panting mess in order for it to be effective or worth my time. Subconsciously, I think a part of me even believed it would be doubly effective if I woke up at 5am to do it. It wasn't, it just made me really tired, and this early morning motivation never lasted much more than a week or two before I would give up. I guess you could say I was following a 'no pain, no gain' mantra, a fairly toxic message that probably still lurks in the back of most of our minds when we think of exercise. If you enjoy pushing yourself to the limit with every workout, then more power to you. But for those of us who just want to be a little healthier and maybe in slightly better shape, I think this ethos around exercise can do more harm than good. Especially when we're just starting out. I don't believe that becoming healthier, or improving general mobility, requires anything drastic or ridiculously intense, I think it just needs consistency.

Don't get me wrong, I'm all for a challenge. And throughout the book I'm going to encourage you to step out of your comfort zone into movement and mindset territories you've never walked before. But it's important you do it at your own pace, and that you learn to shift gears and develop an understanding of when to push and when to pull back on the intensity, rather than running at everything as fast as possible. In fact, if you're attempting to approach exercise with this million-miles-an-hour mentality, you're more likely to end up burning out and injured, which doesn't lend itself to the idea of maintaining consistency. The wonderful news is how little exercise you actually need to do in order to reap the rewards.

Minimal Effective Dose

The concept of a minimal effective dose is something I wish I'd grasped a lot sooner. The idea is to do as little as possible and still get results – sounds appealing, right? Well, maybe not as little as possible, but 'just enough' to get results. If you want to improve your health, but struggle to maintain consistent exercise habits, I need you to know that you don't need to overhaul your life to reap at least some of the good stuff. As consistency is a core concept of building a body that lasts (and success in life in general), finding an amount of work you can genuinely stick to over a longer period of time will lead to better long-term results than doing as much as possible for two weeks and then never again.

This doesn't mean we won't push it every now and again, or that frequent, intense exercise is necessarily a bad thing – far from it. Frequent and more intense exercise absolutely has a time and a place, but it doesn't need to be *all the time*. There is definitely such a thing as too much, too quickly, especially if you're new to exercise or you struggle to maintain consistency.

So, how much exercise do you actually need to do to start bringing home the rewards? A 'meta-analysis' (a fancy way of saying a study that includes lots of other studies) conducted in 2022 suggests that just 60 minutes of lifting weights per week is enough to reduce your risk of all causes of death by up to 27 per cent, while even just engaging in any resistance training at all resulted in a 15 per cent reduced risk when compared with none at all[1]. So just one hour a week and you'll have reduced your chance of death by about a third. That's 30 minutes twice a week, or less than 10 minutes a day – I'll let that sink in. The same research also suggests those who engage in a combination of both cardio-based activities and resistance training see a 46 per cent lower risk of developing cardiovascular disease.

But what about flexibility? Surely we need to be slogging it more than this to get bendier? Apparently not. The research we have suggests that 5 minutes of stretching, per movement, per week, is enough to improve flexibility substantially.[2] Most benefit is experienced when this movement is spread throughout a week, rather than all on one day, with the greatest improvements seen when it's broken down into 30-second stretches. Simply put, that's 10 x 30 seconds, which could be twice a day, five days a week. Neat, huh?

On the strength side, expert opinion currently agrees that one to three heavy sets of weightlifting, one to three times a week, will produce significant strength improvements.[3]

I'm not suggesting that doing more physical activity than this minimal recommended dose is a waste of time. It's no secret that most of us could benefit from more exercise, and that aiming for more than the minimal dose will doubtless lead to greater benefits. That being said, you don't have to kill yourself in order to milk the rewards of exercise, and even a smidge can have a massive impact, especially if it means you'll actually keep up with it in the long term. Despite being one of the greatest songs of all time, it pains me to say that when it comes to exercise, Luther Vandross got it wrong – there really is such a thing as too much.

The Goldilocks Zone

If you're desperate to improve your health but find it impossible to stick to an exercise routine and build consistent movement habits, it's time to focus on doing less and building up gradually over time. While I'm not actually recommending doing as little as physically possible (i.e. nothing) aiming for a smaller, but still effective amount, rather than a maximal dose, may just be the necessary remedy you need to reap the rewards of exercise more sustainably. *How to Build a Body That Lasts* is about finding your personal sweet spot, your Goldilocks Zone, which ultimately will look different for everyone. If you love exercise and you're in a consistent groove already, that is amazing. If you have the habits down but want some tips and tricks to improve your joint health, there's plenty of that to come. But if you don't love exercise, or you're struggling to stick to a consistent routine, or maybe you keep picking up injuries, you don't have to kill yourself to make positive changes.

I want to start by shifting the focus away from how much *can* you do, towards this 'Goldilocks' approach, where you strive to do *just enough* and build up over time. And finding what the right amount looks like for you personally is about trial and error.

CHANGE PLACES

I think it's about time we got a wiggle on, don't you?

All I need you to do now is *change position.*

This might mean standing up and changing seats, or simply having a little shuffle on your bum to change the position of your body. Whatever you do – move.

To be clear, there's nothing wrong with sitting down, and if I've caught you hunched over this book like a prawn, or lying like a croissant, there's no need to sit bolt upright. There's little evidence to suggest that any *one* posture or position is better than another, but when it comes to battling chronic stiffness, pain and improving your mobility, it's important that you move, and move often.[4]

There is an entire chapter later in the book dedicated to posture, so if you do want to know more, stick around. For now, I just want you to move, and every time you see the words CHANGE PLACES throughout the book, use my little nag as a reminder to have a shuffle, a little rearrange, and keep that body rolling so it doesn't spend too long in any one position.

While we're at it. I also want to remind you to BREATHE. Use this little break to take a big ol' breath and get those lungs expanding while you're having a shimmy. All done? Great. Now get nice and comfy before we move on to the next chapter.

Wiggle Week

If you've come to this book looking for a quick plan to improve your mobility, then this is the chapter for you. But before I get you rolling around your living room and challenge your movement abilities in all kinds of weird and wonderful ways, I want to share some sensationally simple mobility-moulding nuggets that you can implement into your life *today.* Welcome to Wiggle Week.

Every day this week I want you to challenge yourself to incorporate a different movement into your day.

> Day 1: Balance on one leg while you brush your teeth. Set a timer for 2 minutes and try to balance for 1 minute on each leg. Don't worry if you can't manage a whole minute, just challenge yourself to avoid dropping your lifted foot as few times as possible!
>
> Day 2: Sit on the floor for 20 minutes. While watching TV, scrolling on your phone, sending emails, or simply enjoying some down time, get your butt on the floor for at least 20 minutes. I don't care how you sit – the more you move, shuffle and wiggle about, the better. This is an amazing way of getting some good stretching into your hips.
>
> Day 3: Go for a walk. You can call a friend, listen to a podcast, be at one with nature – but whatever you do, strut your stuff! It doesn't matter how long (to be fair, probably more than 5 minutes, but I'm not here

to judge) how far, or how fast you walk. All I care about is that you get outside for a designated walk and stomp those feet.

Day 4: Perform countertop push ups every time the kettle boils or you make a meal. Making a cuppa? Do some push ups on the countertop! Making a sandwich? Do some push ups on the countertop! Using the microwave? Do some push ups on the countertop! You get the idea. Doesn't matter how many, just place those hands on the countertop, lower your chest down, push up, and repeat as many times as you can throughout the day. If you're proficient in floor-based push ups, don't let me hold you back – go wild. The important thing is that you push it real good.

Day 5: Squat every time you open the fridge. Next time you whip that fridge door open, it's time to do some squats – 1, 5 or 10 – however many squats you like! The rule is: when the fridge pops, you drop it like it's hot.

Day 6: Sleep: Go to bed 1 hour (or even 30 minutes) earlier (if possible). Rest and recovery is everything when it comes to a mobile body, so if it's humanly possible, get yourself to sleep earlier tonight. If you have young kids or a job that doesn't allow you to get extra Zs, limit your screen time before bed instead.

Day 7: Do something you *love*. Happiness and healthiness go hand in hand, so whatever you do today, do something positive for yourself – literally anything that's going to put a smile on your face and bring you genuine joy. This doesn't have to be a 'health seeking behaviour' specifically, it can even be a little indulgent, whatever it is, just make sure it's something that you really love.

I'm not suggesting that you have to abide by these seven commandments in order to waltz through the pearly gates of mobility heaven. Nor am I saying there's no need to read the rest of this book. But sometimes we just don't have the time to commit 100 per cent, even when we know it's good for us. So the Wiggle Week challenge is a simple seven-day approach to help springboard your mobility efforts and get you moving more, even when time and energy levels are super tight.

The challenge here is to be consistent in doing *something,* rather than consistently doing *nothing.* You can carry these movements through more than one day, adding each one to your hand until you build an entire deck of wiggles that you can shuffle seamlessly into your life, and if you're feeling really spicy, you can even make up your own. Whatever you do, I want you to make a pledge that this week is Wiggle Week, and thou shalt Wiggle – got it?

Mobility Snacks

You don't stop playing because you grow old, you grow old because you stop playing.

(George Bernard Shaw – no idea who he is, but I like the quote)

Dedicated, structured mobility sessions are a sensational way of improving your abilities, and a key part of this book, but as you'll see during your Wiggle Week, they ain't the only tool in the toolbox. If you *really* want to improve how you move and make it last, it helps to take a two-pronged attack and sprinkle movement across your day as regularly and often as possible. Rather than relying solely on the benefits of a few workouts here or there throughout the week, maximise your movement time during your daily life. Start with the Wiggle Week, then begin to introduce more and more 'Mobility Snacks' throughout your day.

If you're anything like me and you find yourself randomly opening the fridge 30 times a day, you'll be very familiar with snacks. While a mobility snack isn't quite as delicious, these little nuggets of movement can have a monumentally positive impact on your health and wellbeing over time as you consistently introduce them into your life.

You've probably heard someone somewhere spout some unhelpful rubbish along the lines of 'We all have the same 24 hours in a day' when it comes to exercising. The issue I have with this short-sighted idea is that although the sands of time may fall the same for all of us, the demands on each of us within those 24 hours are drastically different. I don't think shouting or guilting anyone into exercise is a helpful approach, especially those who are already struggling to juggle an endless list of tasks. We all know that we need to move more – it doesn't mean we need to do five killer workouts every week. Instead, we need to shift the focus away from an 'all or nothing' mindset towards a 'something is always better than nothing' approach, and this is where our Mobility Snacks come in.

Simply put, a Mobility Snack is a short burst of movement, which, when spread throughout the day, helps create a more accessible approach to movement, especially when dedicated exercise feels totally out of reach. This bite-sized approach helps us 'sneak' these snacks into our life and bank our movement minutes each day, which can be extra handy for those gruelling times – either at work or at home – when we simply can't face the idea of a full workout. They allow us to contribute to our movement quota and keep the movement juices flowing, even when time is short.

Here are a few examples of Mobility Snacks you can play around with:

- Balance on one leg while brushing your teeth.
- Push ups on the countertop while you boil the kettle.
- Squats when you open the fridge.
- Deep squat hold while you wait for the microwave.
- Elephant walk while you read an email (page 76).
- Couch stretch when you sit down to watch the TV (page 114).
- Calf raises when you walk up the stairs.
- Jumping on the spot while you wait for a train (even if it looks funny).

Doing five squats when you open the fridge and five push ups when you boil the kettle probably doesn't sound like a lot, and really that's the point – it shouldn't feel like a lot, it should feel doable. The real benefit isn't in the immediate action but the compound interest over time, when you stack these movements alongside things you do a lot throughout the day. By the time you've opened the fridge or had your sixth cup of tea of the day, you've squeezed in 30 squats and 30 push ups without dedicating any extra time to movement outside of what you're already doing.

That's 210 squats a week.
That's 910 a month.
That's 10,950 a year.

Suddenly your cute little five squats and five push ups here and there rack up to over 10,000 a year, and *that*, my wonderful friend, is where the impact really lies. I guarantee that if you repeat a movement 10,000 times in a year you'll be blown away by the improvement in your movement snacks of choice, but also your health and overall wellbeing. And even if you only stuck to this 50 per cent of the time, that's still 5,000 squats and push ups in a year – that's *a lot* of movement. Compare this to doing 30 squats in a workout three times a week (90 squats), or absolutely nothing at all, and hopefully you can start to see how these tiny little snacks can be so beneficial.

Don't get me wrong – I still want you to find space for dedicated movement practices that fit into your life; these more systematic sessions are our bread and butter. But the real mobility magic amplifies when we combine the approaches of dedicated training sessions that fit our schedule, with everyday movement 'snacks'. The most important thing is that you take this at your own pace but challenge yourself to seize more movement opportunities.

To really make this concept stick, the idea is to pair a movement with something you already do regularly. You may be familiar with a concept known as 'habit stacking', which is a sensational tool to help develop new routines. Rather than relying solely on our ability to remember to move (which is hard enough at the best of times in our busy lives), we latch a new, good habit on to something we do regularly and which is well established in our day to act as a reminder. It may also help to prompt yourself with a Post-It note somewhere prominent as well!

Don't just rely on my suggestions for Mobility Snack ideas; nobody knows your life better than you, so get creative and think about where you can wiggle some snacks in. And if you find one of the movement challenges in this book hits the spot for you, consider where you can sprinkle that snack into your day.

Challenge: Think of three things you do regularly throughout your day and three movements you can pair them with. Pop a Post-It where this activity goes down as a reminder and get to it!

What Do You Want?

This chapter is arguably the most important part of *How to Build a Body That Lasts*. I know we haven't started moving much yet, but before we do it's a good idea to know *why* you're doing it in the first place. Beyond the obvious physical benefits, it's key to know why it's important to *you*. What you need to really uncover is how improving your mobility will improve your own life, and what that means to you as a unique human being. In other words, your mobility hopes, dreams and purpose.

Wanting to learn the splits is all well and good, and I'd be lying if I said I wouldn't love to show off and bust them out at every possible opportunity, but the truth is I've gotten through 30 years of life just fine without ever needing to do the splits, or even coming close. None of this is to say there isn't benefit in mastering a difficult physical skill – there's plenty. But most of us don't need *extreme* levels of mobility; just to be able to go about life and do the things we love without feeling as though we're fighting a battle with our body.

If the reason for wanting to learn the splits is to show off your shiny new skills, then I love that and I'm here for it. But be aware that there's a strong possibility your *why* may not be strong enough to carry you there, without the risk of your motivation dropping off the face of a cliff. If you compare it with other, more internal motivations, like wanting to maintain the ability to get up from the floor with ease, or to play with your kids and grand-kids, or to overcome pain in your hip so you can get back to the sport you love . . . now those are powerful whys, because they're important to *you*.

It might just be that you want to feel a little better in yourself – this is enough of a reason to get started. However, if you want this movement malarkey to stick, to become embedded into your life as a habit for the long run, then knowing *why* you want to improve how you move is job number one.

Don't worry if you have no idea yet – that's what we're about to work out.

Grab a pen and paper, or even your phone. It's question time, and I want you to scribble your own answers.

Before you start note-taking, please remember that this is about what *you* want, and nobody else. Be as detailed as possible and take as much time as you need, but be sure to be wholeheartedly honest with what *you* want. No matter how big or small, how silly or serious it may seem, this is a safe space to explore your movement hopes and dreams.

Let's start with these three questions:

Why is mobility important to you?
Which benefits of improving your mobility matter the most to you?
How will these improvements in your mobility make your life better?

Don't panic if you're drawing a blank and can't think of anything. It's totally normal not to know the answer yet, but I at least want you to start thinking about it. Sleep on it and come back to this another day. Whatever you do, be honest with yourself. It may help to think of something you love or have always wanted to do. What part does your mobility play in your ability to do that thing? This is where you should start.

If you ever start to feel a little demotivated (which is completely normal), you can look back at your list and remind yourself why you started in the first place. This is an incredibly simple yet powerful way of giving yourself a kick up the bum to get going again.

My Why

At the time of writing, my pending baby daughter has been cooking for 20 weeks and rapidly developing in her mum's tum. It feels wild to think that by the time you're reading this I'll be a dad to a tiny human. I still feel like a big child myself; the voice in my head still feels the same as when I was 17, and I'll probably be saying the same thing when I'm 70. As my daughter rockets into existence, I find myself both in awe of the life she has ahead of her, but also loudly recognising the finitude of mine. This might sound a little bleak, talking about death at the ripe old age of 30, but that's far from my intention, and I don't think it has to be bleak at all. If anything, I think that acknowledging and revelling in the fact that we only get one of these bodies, for a limited amount of time, is the single greatest motivator to appreciate it while we can. That being said, I haven't always felt this way, or paid much attention to my health or wellbeing.

Like most of us, in my late teens and early twenties I thought I was invincible. The last thing on my mind was my health. I'd always been an active kid, from rugby to volleyball to cricket to skateboarding, and I loved it. But I didn't ever actively think about fitness – I just liked chasing balls around. PE was the only subject in school that sparked any interest in me, so much so that I enrolled at the University of Leeds to study sports and exercise science with the eventual aim of becoming a PE teacher. I went to university with every intention of joining sports clubs, but when I arrived I suddenly felt incredibly intimidated by the idea. Despite having played rugby for the last eight years, I felt I wasn't big enough, strong enough, or enough of a 'rugby lad' to get involved. I dabbled with volleyball and the occasional game of five-aside football, but my love for sport had begun to wane and instead I found myself deep in the nightlife of Leeds.

I'm not proud of this chapter of my life: I smoked, drank far too much, and took an excessive number of illicit substances. I regularly stayed up for 40+ hours at a time, and my diet was horrendous, as I would rather spend money on partying than food. Looking back, I don't recognise this version of myself, and I didn't realise at the time that my mental health was *low* (surprise, surprise).

I tried to kickstart my health a few times throughout my uni years. The problem is that health isn't a lawnmower and doesn't respond to kickstarting. Your health is more like a garden where seeds need to be planted, watered and given time to grow, consistently nourished with TLC. At one point, I even started going to the gym in my attempt to clean up my act. Well, I went once, only to dislocate my shoulder trying to lift the same amount as my friend, Archie, who was a lot stronger than me. It felt as though the world was telling me, 'Exercise isn't for you, Adam,' and I believed it. I was studying a sports science degree, applying none of it to my life, and I felt like a fraud.

So how did I go from regularly abusing my body to writing a book about how to take care of it?

One Saturday night in June 2015, three days before my last ever university exam, I'd just watched *Mad Max* (the one with Mel Gibson, not Tom Hardy) with my housemates and gone to bed. I woke up at 2am with a headache like I'd never had before. I crept into my housemate Steph's bedroom to steal some paracetamol and tried to go back to sleep, and that's the last I remember. My brother lived with me at the time and had gone out for the night. When he stumbled home at 6am, he heard me stomping around in my bedroom. A little shocked I was even awake at that time, he walked up to my room to find me delirious, eyes rolling in the back of my head, stumbling about my bedroom, unrecognisable and spouting absolute gibberish. He called the paramedics, and they whisked me off to A&E, where they confirmed I had contracted bacterial meningitis. Meningitis is an infection that causes the outer layer of your brain, known as your meninges, to swell. There are two types of meningitis: viral, which your body can fight off by itself, and bacterial, which requires antibiotics. If left untreated, this infection can lead to an array of complications including hearing loss, vision loss, limb loss, coordination and balance problems, and in 10 per cent of cases, death.

I spent the next three days in an induced coma, waking up on Tuesday afternoon in intensive care, surrounded by my family, not having a clue what the hell had just happened. My brother didn't leave my bedside for that whole time, and if he hadn't been there and hadn't bothered to check on me, I can confidently say I wouldn't be here now (thank you, Alec). Thanks to how swiftly everyone involved reacted, I woke up without so much as a scratch on me. I'd love to tell you that this 'near-death experience' acted as a catalyst for me to seize the day, grab my life and health by the nuts and embark on a journey of self-discovery. It did not. I basically just had a really long nap and 12 days later decided to go to a festival in Barcelona. I carried on smoking, partying and eating very little, and this is when my mental and physical health really plummeted.

Five months later and I got meningitis again. Who knew you could get it twice? I certainly did not. The second time was much worse; there was no long nap, and I was awake and conscious for the whole thing. Steph came home from a lecture to find me curled up on the sofa and rushed me to the doctors. I'll never forget the look on the nurse's face when she saw me stumble in. She rushed me past everyone else and dragged me upstairs without hesitation, where she took my temperature and called an ambulance immediately. Following the insertion of a big needle in my spine known as a lumbar puncture, it was confirmed: bacterial meningitis round two. After four days of a pounding headache, I have a newfound empathy for anyone who deals with migraines, and now every time I get even the suggestion of a sore head, I instinctively put my chin to my chest to hopefully rule out round three. If you're wondering what I'm waffling on about here, one of the symptoms of meningitis is a stiff neck, caused by the swelling to the brain and spinal cord, making it hard or even impossible to touch your chin to your chest.[1] I spent seven days in hospital, but after a lot of drugs, countless blood tests and enough daytime TV for a lifetime, I was allowed to go home. Yet again without a scratch on me, but this time with a growing appreciation for the fact I was alive, with a completely functioning body, and a love for the NHS and the incredible staff of St James's Hospital in Leeds.

I can't help but feel my body was trying to send me a message by slapping me in the face with meningitis twice. It would be naive for me to suggest that people bring sickness or misfortune upon themselves intentionally through how they act. Accidents happen, and genetics plays an incredibly influential role in who develops sickness and disease, and that's nobody's fault. However, as the guardian of my own body, I believe I have to accept a certain level of responsibility for how I care for my magical meat suit (aka my home). I believe the body is phenomenal at giving us feedback, and that if something in our body doesn't feel right, it's our job to listen to it the best we can; for me, in that moment, it very much felt like my body was trying to tell me something.

I know there will be some of you who weren't as lucky as I was, who did walk away with scars, and of course there will be others who didn't have the fortune to walk away at all. I don't want to preach to you about how you live your life. It's *your* life. I just wholeheartedly hope that you decide to make the most of what's important to you, while you can. Now more than ever, I want to live in one relatively well-functioning body and enjoy as much of life as I can with my little baby girl and the love of my life.

Now, don't get me wrong. It wasn't as if I just jumped out of hospital straight into the gym on a mission to sculpt an indestructible body. Far from it. And meningitis wasn't my only motivator. As I mentioned, if you had asked me a few years ago why I started exercising again, despite all my health ups and downs, I would have told you that it was to grow some muscle and to become sexier. A cliché, I know. But back then, I didn't like the way I looked and wanted to change it. So I started going to the gym and lifting weights.

Fast-forward a few years into my 'get sexy' gym mission and, following countless cycles of starting and stopping, and failing to make exercise a consistent habit, I guess I am finally 'there'. I always found myself coming back eventually, because every time I exercised, I felt better. So after years of half-hearted efforts, even though I still hadn't quite nailed the consistency part, exercise started to become a more regular feature in my life. And although becoming sexier was still high on my list, my priorities really started to shift away from just how I *looked* and more towards how my body *felt*.

Exercise simply made my brain feel good – but the way I was exercising made my body feel beaten up, and it seemed like every time I recovered from an injury, I picked up another one. I was learning the hard way that I was doing too much too quickly, not giving my body a chance to adapt and picking up injuries as a result of my impatience. I wanted to be able to trust my body, but to do that I had to respect it, too. Yet as I tried to listen to my body, it was as if we were speaking different languages – and it was at this point that I dived down the rabbit hole of mobility.

My relationship with my body is on an ongoing rollercoaster of love, with the inevitable ups and downs. But I've finally started to feel as if my body and I speak the same language, that we understand each other better than ever (although I do still get it wrong from time to time). This epiphany has been so life-changing for me that I want to help you understand how to do the same with your body, and how to fulfil your own personal purpose.

My *why* has evolved over the years, and I'm sure yours will too. Hitting an all-time low health-wise, along with my mission to become sexier, got me started, but it was the desire to feel good that kept me going. Dedicating time to listening, understanding and working with my body to improve how I move has been invaluable. Now when I consider my *why,* as I hurtle towards parenthood, I can't help but feel an overwhelming sense of the importance of being able to move with freedom, and an appreciation of how blink-and-you'll-miss-it life truly is. I want to be able to play with my daughter, and to care for her and my partner for as long as possible.

I'm not expecting my story to motivate you to work on your mobility. But I'd bet my kneecaps that there is *somebody* or *something* out there that makes your life worth living. I wonder if you've ever stopped to think about why keeping mobile and healthy in both body and soul might be important to you. What are the things or who are the people that make life worth living? What makes movement important to you?

We're all social creatures at heart, and a sense of community is important to our wellbeing as humans. Sometimes doing stuff for yourself can be difficult, but when you have a purpose beyond just yourself, it can help ignite that spark you needed all along. Whether it's your best friend, your partner, your sister, your son or daughter, your grandparent, your ping-pong partner, your cat, your dog or your frog – remembering who's important to you can be a poignant reminder to help take care of yourself when you need it the most.

What Does Success Even Mean?

When I first started working as a personal trainer, one of my first ever clients, Zara, asked me, 'What is your definition of success?'

She metaphorically slapped me round the mush with one of the most profound questions I've ever been asked, and one I've asked every person I've ever worked with since. I want to ask you the same thing, but with a fruity little topical twist.

What does healthy and fit look like to you?

Don't worry if you're drawing a blank – that's okay! It took me a while to work it out too. Take some time to sit and think about it, but remember that this is about what fitness looks like to *you*, and nobody else. The reason I'm banging on about all this aims and objectives stuff is because the last thing I want is for you to spend any more of your precious time or energy climbing up your ladder of health and fitness success, only to find that the ladder was on the wrong wall the whole time. There's an incredible amount of noise in the world of health and fitness, and despite what the media has portrayed since the dawn of time, I passionately believe that you don't need to have rippling muscles, be super lean, sensationally strong or even wildly flexible to be healthy and to live a fulfilling life.

As I've spoken about, when I was starting out, I believed that looking a certain way would make me happy. It didn't. I'll say this right now: health and fitness don't have a 'look'. But they definitely have a feel, and a big part of finding your 'feel' is down to pursuing what's important to you. Knowing your definition of success is the best way to prevent getting dragged along someone else's path of health and fitness – even mine. So this is why I think it's worth doing some digging and working out what's important to you, and that all starts with how you define success.

Think about what you really want to get out of your body. The answer to this question is ultimately the North Star. Look at it often and embody it through what you do.

You've shown me yours, so it's only fair I show you mine.

My definition of success is: *Progress in the right direction, irrespective of speed.*

I've sat with this definition for quite some time now, and it's become a value of mine that has shaped my approach to fitness. It's allowed me to remove a lot of external pressure from my life by putting things into perspective, especially when it comes to what *I* perceive as fitness versus what I see on social media. At the heart of it all, it's about doing my best to keep chipping away like a little woodpecker and making tiny bits of progress, irrespective of how quickly I get there. Life can sometimes feel like a constant quest to be as productive as possible, to optimise everything, and that can leave you with a constant feeling of unease; that no matter how much you're doing, you're just not doing enough. I'm not saying my mantra stops that feeling completely – I don't think it'll ever truly go away. But it gives me a framework, an anchor with which to settle myself down and bring myself back to reality.

When I focus on the progress I've made, it gives me a reference point for how far I've come. The ability to look back at where I once was in comparison to where I am now has helped me overcome so much of my internal angst. When I find myself drifting into a sea of comparison, staring in front of me at the things I want to achieve or don't have, my anchor helps pull me back to a place where I can appreciate how far I've already come, rather than how far I have to go. It also helps keep my sight on my next step: becoming a slightly better me.

This doesn't mean I'm progressing all the time, every second of every day, or even that I won't go backwards at points. Progress doesn't happen in a straight line and setbacks are inevitable. But it does mean that when I face a setback, I'm able to focus on the small positive steps that keep me travelling in the right direction. Irrespective of how long it takes me, as long as I'm moving forwards, in my eyes, I'm succeeding.

I hope you're starting to get a better idea of why you want to get moving in the first place. In the next chapter we'll look at how you can track your mobility progress to help you keep moving in the right direction!

Time to Move

Welcome to the movement challenge section! I hope you're ready to get wiggling. After all, we're not just here to talk about mobility. Although I firmly believe the previous chapters play an integral part in framing how you and I will approach this section of the book (and maybe even life in general), talking will only take us so far. Improving your mobility is a bit like juggling: no matter how much you talk about it, the only way you're going to get better is to grab it by the balls and do it again and again and again.

In this part of the book, we're going to assess how you move, but please know that this section isn't a 'test' with a pass or fail mark at the end. I have no intention of sparking any school-based PTSD. Instead, we are going to dabble through 20 different movement challenges, aimed at testing your balance, strength and flexibility in a variety of positions (think Kama Sutra without the sex) to better understand what your body can do physically. I want to be clear that these movements aren't 'gold standards' or 'musts' in order to thrive and live a good life. They're simply a series of challenges to objectively measure (without judgement) and identify what you're physically capable of and what you struggle with at this current moment in time, while equipping you with plenty of exercises to build into your movement port-folio. We will also explore why these specific movements may be important to you and how they might relate to your day-to-day life and overall wellbeing. Once we know where you are now, we can look at where to go next and how to shuffle these moves into your life.

At the beginning of each challenge I'll point out which body parts you'll be using and what your body is about to do, while teaching you the meaning of some basic movement lingo, like flexion and extension, to help you better understand what's going on at each joint and which muscles you'll be targeting with each move. In this case, flexion and extension are two words used to describe movement around a joint in which the angle gets smaller or larger. Think about someone flexing their arms to show off their biceps (guns): the angle at the elbow gets smaller. When the arm is extended, the angle gets bigger. Learning the basics of this seemingly fancy movement language as we work through these challenges will help set you up for mobility success, ready to spread your wings beyond this book into the big bad exercise world, better equipped to know what us fitness lot are waffling on about when describing movement.

Some of these movement challenges might be easy, while some might feel really tough and maybe even a little uncomfortable, but nothing we're about to do should hurt. There's a big difference between discomfort and pain, but that line can feel very fine, especially when you don't have too much experience. A bit of discomfort is to be expected when we're challenging our body and doing things we've never done before, but if any of these movements do cause you pain, there will be exercise adaptations for you to try, and an entire chapter dedicated to teaching you how to navigate painful movements and make them work for you. At no point throughout these challenges should you be working through excessive pain. Instead, we want to learn how to adapt these movements so we can keep chipping away and making progress without agony.

Tracking Progress

To help set you up for mobility success, it essential to track your progress. This is going to help maintain motivation, but more importantly show you you're headed in the right direction. Here are three simple ways to track your pending mobility world domination.

Adam's 1–10 Scoring System

Firstly, while you're getting your wiggle on throughout these challenges, pay attention as you move. Give the movement a difficulty rating out of 10. To keep this nice and simple, 1= *Easy* and 10 = *Wow, that's actually impossible, I might explode.*

I appreciate this isn't the clearest of difficulty scales, so here's a little more detail to help guide you.

1 = SO easy, I'm practically laying down in bed.
2 = Still easy, I could do this all day.
3 = I can start to feel it, but this is still an absolute breeze.
4 = Ooh, I think I can feel it now. It's still manageable and I'd have no problem doing this for a long time. But, yeah, I'm aware of it.
5 = I can definitely feel the difficulty increasing! This is mildly challenging.
6 = More than mildly challenging and I can really feel it now. But I could keep going at this intensity for a while. And I can keep up a slow conversation while doing this.
7 = It just got a little spicy in here – did someone turn up the heat? I'm still in control, but I feel challenged and this is getting hard! I can talk, but I need to focus.

8 = *Wawaweewa, this is tough! This is the highest level of
intensity I can maintain with control for any length of time.
I can just about talk but you're not getting much from me
other than a few words.*

9 = *Oh hot damn! I can't keep this up. Any harder and I feel like
I might injure myself! I can't speak while doing this.*

10 = *I literally could not work any harder or bear any more if I
tried. Am I dying?*

Don't worry too much about being super specific or getting the rating 'wrong'; this is a made-up system designed to encourage you to pay attention to how your body feels, and to listen and adjust accordingly. It doesn't have to be super accurate or objective.

When you first start asking yourself to identify how hard something is out of 10, it's likely going to feel as though you're pulling an arbitrary number out of the air, and that's okay. The more you move and the more you ask yourself this question, the better the relationship between you and your body will become and the more accurate you'll become at deciphering how hard something is on your personal difficulty scale.

You may have heard of this scoring system referred to as an 'RPE' scale, meaning Rate of Perceived Exertion. But as it's a scale personal to you, you can call it whatever you want!

Take Note

Secondly, to spice things up a little and make your efforts even more effective, I want to encourage you to take note of what you feel and where you feel the discomfort. Feel stiff in your hips? Take a note! Sharp pain in your shoulder when you lift it above your head? Take a note! Feel easy on the left side but tight on the right? Take a note! The more notes you take, the better. Each movement challenge will include prompts for you to think about while you wiggle, but the main thing is to pay attention, listen to your body and write it down.

This will help in a couple of ways:

1. These challenges aren't a one-time rodeo. They're here for you to come back to at any point to see your improvement. I guarantee after a month of busting these moves, you won't remember how they felt the very first time you did them. Having a rating out of 10 and some simple notes such as 'Wowee, right groin felt super tight, can't get elbow anywhere near the floor. 8/10', will work wonders for seeing how you've improved. Paying attention to how things feel in the moment will pay dividends in the future when you get that kick of progress dopamine. When you're saying 'Oh hot damn, that's much easier now. Groin feels way looser and my elbow is on the floor! 5/10', you'll be so glad you charted where you started. High five to you!

2. Learning to speak the language of your body takes time and repetition, but it gets better a lot faster when you actually listen to one another. Observing how you feel, paying attention while you move, and writing it all down will fast-track you to developing better bodily awareness, which is key to mastering your mobility.

Consider this part of your 'progress journal', an opportunity for you to look back with a smile of pride at how you once found something difficult that now feels a breeze . . .

Whip Out Your Camera!

Your camera is going to be your best friend when it comes to tracking your mobility progress. Over time, as you get bendier, stronger, more supple, stable and coordinated, you might not notice the subtle differences, but when you look back and compare images or videos side by side, you'll see so much improvement (if you put in the practice, of course). This is invaluable for keeping motivation high. Throughout the challenges, I'm going to remind you to whip out your camera and film yourself. You don't need Spielberg levels of production here, just prop a camera against a wall or water bottle so it can see you. And you don't have to do anything with your footage if you don't want to, but if you do want to share it with the world, post it on social media with #HowToBuildABodyThatLasts. We can inspire an army of bendy humans and I can give you my personal feedback!

Enough waffle, it's time to move.

But first, let's all CHANGE PLACES and take a nice BREATH. Ooooweee, I needed that.

Flamingo Disco: Balance

Ideal for: Feet, Ankles, Knees, Hips
and Core Muscle Stability

Welcome to the most underrated aspect of fitness. When was the last time you thought about your balance? The beauty of balance is that on a day-to-day level, we don't need to focus on it too much; our body does that for us. For this challenge, however, we're going to bring our balance to the forefront of our minds to see if it's up to scratch. Just make sure you're next to something soft, like a bed or a sofa, because we're going to find out how gravity is really treating you.

Before we start, this is your gentle reminder to WHIP OUT YOUR CAMERA and record yourself.

CHALLENGE ONE: SINGLE-LEG BALANCE

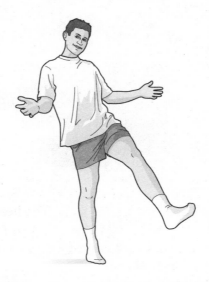

Stand on one leg and time how long you can balance for without putting the other foot down. When your other foot touches the ground, that's your time!

CHALLENGE TWO: CLOSED EYES BALANCE

Do it again – but this time with your eyes closed.

If you want to make Challenges One and Two a little spicier, lift your heel off the ground and stand on your tip toes. This is a great way to challenge the strength of your feet.

CHALLENGE THREE: THE OLD MAN TEST

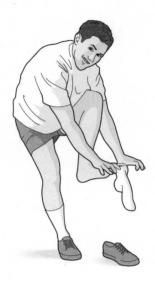

Start standing, with bare feet, and put your sock and then shoe on your foot while balancing on the other leg. Do not let your sock and shoe foot touch the ground. Once you've successfully shoed and socked one foot, hop onto the other leg and do the same on the other side. This is known in rather old-fashioned language as 'The Old Man Test', but no matter your age or gender, it's a good one.

Ideally, you want to build up to being able to balance on one leg for more than 30 seconds on each side with both eyes open and then eyes closed, and pass The Old Man Test without falling over. If you're worried about falling, set up next to something you can hold on to, like a wall or door frame, to support you. Gently let go and see how long you can last without any extra support.

Top tip: Take big, slow breaths and focus on squeezing your glutes (bum cheeks) and keeping your core nice and tight. This will help keep you stable. Don't be afraid to use your arms to counterbalance. As you get better at balancing, you'll need your arms less and less!

TAKE NOTE

- Rate the difficulty 1–10 for Challenges One, Two and Three.
- How long did you manage?
- Were you wobbly or did you feel nice and steady?
- Could you feel the muscles in your feet and ankles working?
- How about your glutes and core muscles?
- Did you notice any difference between your left and right side?

Wobbling All Over the Shop?

If you struggled to balance for more than 30 seconds on either leg with your eyes open, then this section is for you. If you sailed through the first challenge but fell short once your vision was taken out of the equation in Challenge Two, or once movement was added in The Old Man Test, then you have a decent base balance and with a little more practice you'll be showing off your stability in no time.

If you found one side a lot easier than the other, that's completely normal. Most of us have one dominant side that's stronger and more coordinated. Even if your balance is a little off on one side, the body can still work harmoniously as you meander through life. If one side felt completely useless compared to the other, practising a little more on the less balanced side will help even you up nicely, but rather than worrying about one side being worse than the other, focus on bettering your balance across the board, on both legs.

If you glided seamlessly beyond the 30 seconds in Challenges One and Two, and whipped your socks and shoes on in The Old Man Test without so much as a minor wobble here or there, we can safely say that balance of yours is tip top – well done. Continue practising to keep your brain and body connection as sharp as possible.

These challenges are more than just ways to assess your balance abilities; they also work beautifully as exercises you can repeat regularly to improve and measure your progress. At the end of this chapter we'll explore how you can sprinkle these movements into your life, and other creative ways to help balance practice become embedded as an enjoyable activity and less of a chore. But before we do, let's talk about why balance is important.

Why is Balance Important and How Does it Work?

It's no surprise that balance is important to us humans; after all, we spend a large proportion of our lives frolicking around on two feet, and that wouldn't be possible without our best bud balance. But how does the body actually manage to keep us upright and stop us falling flat on our face day after day?

The brain unifies our senses to create one picture of the world around us. Information through all of our other senses is digested and computed by our brain, seemingly automatically and almost instantaneously, without us needing to bat much of an eyelid. Our brain is constantly assessing in the background, and it's a good job too – if we had to pay attention to everything, life would be a little noisy.

Balance, in particular, relies on feedback through sight; from our muscles, ligaments and tendons through proprioception; and from our ears through our vestibular system. The role our eyes play in balance is apparent if you gave Challenge Two a bash and found yourself wobbling like a big bowl of jelly the moment you closed your eyes. Without our eyes, we have to rely heavily on feedback from our muscles, ligaments and tendons to tell our brain where we are in relation to the world around us; this is known as proprioception.

Proprioception is the body's ability to make sense of where it is, a sort of 'bodily awareness', and is the reason you can walk without having to stare at your feet 24/7. It plays a vital role in our coordination while doing anything and everything. Playing another big part in the balance equation is our vestibular system, which you can find tucked away in the inner ear, working quietly in tandem with proprioception to detect the position and movement of our head through space. This allows us to coordinate our eyes and posture to make sure we stay balanced, also known as equilibrium. Basically, you're an automated information computing machine that's subconsciously working overtime to make sure you don't fall over and hurt yourself. Nice that, ain't it?

This computing system that so lovingly ticks over in the background allows us to complete incredibly complex movements, without much 'active' thought. Think about the last time you took a stroll up some stairs, for example: you probably didn't put much thought into how high the step was, or how far you had to lift your leg, other than perhaps 'these stairs are big'. I'm sure you didn't whack out your trusty measuring tape to ensure you lifted your foot the necessary 9.76cm, did you? You most likely just walked up the stairs while brain and body did the maths for you.

When you consider how much there is for our body to compute, coordinate and control at any one time in terms of individual muscles, bones and joints, just to stop us toppling over, it's miraculous that we're even able to balance in the first place. Let alone maintain that balance while doing incredibly difficult things.

You may have noticed in the challenges above, that in order to stop yourself falling over or putting your foot on the ground, you likely had to flail your arms, your legs, or both. This is a sensational example of how the body automatically problem-solves to keep us balanced, and reveals our incredible ability to correct our position rapidly to keep our centre of gravity where it should be. By simultaneously moving our limbs in all kinds of different directions, the brain is actually working to hold our position. The ability to balance without wobbling all over the place requires our muscles and joints to work in harmony, from the tips of our toes all the way to the top of our head, and you may well feel your muscles working hard in the process, especially around your ankle, glutes and core.

Every time you wobble and attempt to save your balance by making a correction, that's your brain and body getting a little better at working together. The better the connection, the fewer the wobbles.

Getting to this point of 'information automation' doesn't happen overnight, it takes a lot of practice. It may seem like a lifetime ago, but there was a version of you that couldn't balance very well at all. I'm not talking about the last time you were drunk, although this will temporarily throw your vestibular system out of whack.[1] I'm talking about little baby you, fumbling and falling on your bum as you learned to strut your stuff. We spend the early years of our development learning to walk through trial and error and by falling over hundreds of times a day. It's hard to imagine that something that now feels so natural once took all of our brain and body's computing power. Yet as we developed and practised, our brain's neuromuscular connection (a fancy way of saying brain to body connection) became stronger and more in tune, making balancing through our day feel second nature. However, as we start to waltz into the later stages of our life, our brain to body connection begins to wane, our ability to balance starts to waver, and the likelihood of falling becomes a lot higher.[2]

As a bouncy baby only a foot tall, falls are relatively insignificant. But as we become taller and a little less robust in our older age, falls begin to take their toll. Falls are the second biggest cause of accidental death globally, and the biggest cause of injury-related death for anyone over 65.[3] With an ageing population, never before has our ability to stay firm on our own two feet been more important.

Where Should You Start and How Often Should You Practice?

Balance is a skill, and despite this apparent inevitable deterioration as we age, like any other physical skill it's something we can improve by practising, no matter our age. Ideally, the more practice the better but I'm not expecting you to spend the rest of your days like a flamingo. However, if you want to be clicking your heels deep into your golden years, it's a good idea to pay your balance some attention sooner rather than later. In fact, one of the most helpful things for your 'movement pension' is practising your balance.

Unless you have a burning desire to join the circus, practising balance won't require anything drastic, and there's no need to start juggling on a balance ball or slack-lining any time soon (unless you want to!). If you walk a lot and exercise regularly, you're already practising your balance-ability just by living your life. After all, with every step you take, your body has to work to maintain your balance. But if you spend a lot of time sitting at a desk or don't currently exercise much, and you want to keep everything working, sprinkling some dedicated balance practices throughout your life will do wonders for keeping your brain and body connection sharp and reducing the risk of falls as you get older.

The simplest way of tracking your improvement is to time how long you can maintain your balance without having to put your foot down, whether it's with eyes open, eyes closed, or on your tip toes. An improvement in time means your balance is getting better. The other thing to pay attention to is how in control of your body you feel while you're trying to balance – in other words, do you feel less wobbly than when you started?

Putting your shoes and socks on (not in that order) while standing up is one of my favourite ways to practise balance, because it's something almost all of us will do at least once a day, and the most effective practices are those that fit easily into your life. Where you can, challenge yourself to put your socks and shoes on without sitting down; just do it next to your bed so you have a bail-out option if all goes south.

Two of my other favourite times to 'snack' on balance are while I brush my teeth and while the kettle boils. My electric toothbrush runs for two minutes, so it means that both of these activities are time-based and give great feedback on how long I'm able to balance. If you don't have an electric toothbrush but still want feedback, you'll find that as your balance improves, you'll jab yourself in the gums a lot less.

Don't feel you have to follow these examples though. When I lived in London, I used to love getting on the Tube and seeing how long I could go without touching anything to keep me stable. Not only is this a pretty good idea for hygiene reasons, but it allowed me to gamify my journey and make it a little more fun, while also working on my balance. You can also do this on the bus, the train, or any public transport you can stand up on. Just always take care and be ready to grab on to something if you need to so you don't go flying into a stranger's lap.

You know your life better than anyone, so play around and see what and where works best for you, and if you're prone to forget, stick a Post-It note wherever you want to be reminded. Welcome to your new less wobbly life!

Get Low: Squat

*Ideal for: Ankles, Knees,
Hips, Quadriceps, Glutes,
Hamstrings, Adductors,
Calves, Abdominals*

It's time to get your squat on! Go on, do one now, just to see how it looks and feels for you. Don't worry too much if you're not sure how to set up, we'll cover that in plenty of detail soon enough. For now, just do what feels instinctive and sit into your squat slowly and gently. Take at least 3–4 seconds to descend as deep as you can, without any excessive pain. There's no need to drop it like it's hot.

The challenges in this chapter are all variations on this one movement: the squat.

WHIP OUT YOUR CAMERA. You're going to want to record this one.

CHALLENGE ONE: DEEP SQUAT

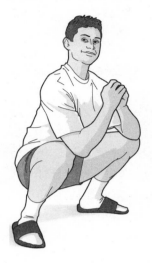

Sit as deep as you can into your squat and see how low you can go with your heels flat on the floor.

Practise a few times until you feel ready for . . .

CHALLENGE TWO: HOW MANY YOU GOT?

Complete as many squats as you can in one go.

Take note of how many you can do and rest for a couple of minutes.

CHALLENGE ONE (*RETEST*)

Now you're a little warmed up, let's retest your deep squat from Challenge One. Time how long you can hold it in the bottom of your squat.

Notice any difference between your first and second deep squat attempt?

What Exactly is a Squat?

If you're unsure what exactly a squat is, imagine you need a poo in the woods but have to keep your trousers on. I know this is a questionable image, but at least you now know what a squat looks like. As you make your way down, if you need to hold on to something for a little stability, that's absolutely fine. Go find a chair, door frame, or anything close by that can provide you with a little support.

TAKE NOTE

- Rate the difficulty 1–10.
- How does it feel down there?
- How low can you go?
- Did you notice a difference in how low you could go in different attempts?
- Can you sit upright or does your torso fall forwards?
- Which way are your feet facing?
- Are your feet flat on the floor or do your heels pop off the ground?
- Any issues? If so, where?
- Pay attention to how your body feels when you're in this position and note exactly where it feels tight or 'not quite right' – the more detail the merrier.

Unlike a lot of personal trainers, I actually don't really care what your squat looks like. I'd love to show you a 'perfect' squat, but I don't believe there is one. All I care about is that you can comfortably sit in a squat position without falling over or feeling like any of your joints are about to explode, then stand back up again with no assistance. There is no specific number of squats you need to be able to do in order to qualify for the Life Olympics (I just made them up), but I think a solid starting point is to be able to complete at least 20 squats without too much pain or feeling like your heart will burst out of your chest. Not only does this demonstrate a bit of strength in your legs but the higher the number, the better the endurance of your leg muscles, and also in your heart, too.

If you struggle to manage just one bodyweight squat, then you've come to the right place. Throughout this chapter we'll explore why mastering this squat is important, but also how you can build up your body's strength so you can drop it with the best of them and show off to everyone in the supermarket when you grace the bottom shelf with your sensational squat.

If you can squat without any trouble but getting to 20 without dying feels out of reach, there's no need to panic. A little more practice and you'll be there in no time.

If you can easily complete 20 – oi oi, big show! It's time to level up and start adding some weight. The easiest way is to buy some at-home dumbbells, kettlebells, a barbell, or a variety of other gym-based equipment, but if you're on a budget, you can get creative and find something with a bit of weight to it, like a backpack stuffed with miscellaneous goods and hold on to it as you make your way through your squats. I'd like to note that you don't have to be able to do 20 squats before you start adding weight. Adding weight is an amazing way of building strength and deepening your squat flexibility as the extra weight helps pull you deeper into the stretch. Some may even find it easier to balance than a bodyweight squat. But if you're getting to 20 unbroken squats and still not adding weight, it's time to challenge yourself. You've got more in the locker, I promise. Just don't feel the need to try and lift as much as you possibly can straight away; start off with a few kilos (or pounds if you're that way inclined) and if that feels too easy, pick up a little more.

Now we know how many squats you can do, how did you get on with the deep squat hold? Spending too long in any position is inevitably going to be uncomfortable. After all, even lying in bed gets uncomfortable after a while, so I'm not expecting you to stay in the squat for ever. But I think a good aim is to be able to hold it for at least a minute or two, ideally longer, without feeling like you're going to expire before standing up again. If you can last longer than a minute, that's a great sign you've got some solid strength in this position.

Can you get low into your squat but struggle to hit the minute mark? No dramas. There's nothing magic about the minute mark, and with a little more practice, you'll nail it anyway. However, if holding this position feels really tough or painful, and the idea of squatting for a minute seems impossible, you could benefit from putting some legwork in here. The simplest way of improving your deep squat is using a little assistance by holding on to something. Over time, as you get stronger down here, you can rely less on external support and more on your own strength.

You may have noticed that your squat looked very different when you first sat into it versus how it looked after you'd repeated the movement a few times. Here's where we introduce a fun fact about your body, and two different 'versions' of your flexibility: cold versus warm. The truth is that you are probably a lot more flexible than you think you are, but when you're at rest, your central nervous system (CNS), responsible for processing all sensory information, prevents you from accessing your full flexible potential as a sort of protective mechanism.

If you were granted full access all the time, you'd more than likely flop about like a cooked noodle and be prone to injury. However, just by exposing your body to a few repetitions of a specific movement and literally warming it up, your central nervous system relaxes a tad, releasing your muscles and connective tissues and allowing them to become a little more elastic. This allows you to access greater range of motion, and for the purposes of this book, we will refer to it as your *warm flexibility*. But – and here's the kicker – after a short while, if you stop making the movement your flexibility will return to its baseline and you will be back in touch with your old friend, *cold flexibility*. The only way to beat this system is by training these positions regularly. The more time we spend in these positions, the more our brain begins to believe they are important to us (practice makes progress, right?). Over time, our CNS starts to trust us a little more, and before you know it, your cold flexibility starts to look a little more like your warm flexibility. If you want to get even more out of your flexibility immediately, make sure you BREATHE into the stretch.

For every flexibility component of these movement challenges, pay attention to your cold versus warm flexibility and, to see progress, compare cold versus cold and warm versus warm over time. Eventually, with practice, your warm flexibility will become your new start point.

How Low Do You Really Need to Go?

If you've read all of this but haven't already got your squat on, what are you waiting for? Stop sitting like a prawn for a minute, bust out a squat and let's see what you've got. If you're still swirling gloriously in your squat while reading this, then well done you lovable show-off; I think it's safe to say you can squat, but the next question is, how low do you really need to go?

There isn't a perfect answer here. You may or may not be familiar with the term 'arse to grass', which is a cheeky little phrase to suggest you should be able to tickle your cheeks with blades of grass when you squat. Instead, a better way of imagining the movement is to get to the point where the backs of your thighs, known as your hamstrings, are able to touch the backs of your shins, known as your calves, with your *whole foot* in contact with the ground. This means no heels popping up. This is often considered to be the 'gold standard' for squats, as it's the furthest possible range of motion any of us will be able to access in this position. However, we're all built differently, and the important thing is that you're aiming to get stronger and more flexible in this position. Focus on improving from wherever you're starting from, getting more comfortable in the position rather than obsessing about how low you can go. If you struggle to get low because of pain, lack of balance, or your heels popping off the floor, let's take a look at a few things that might help you work out why.

To squat successfully, you need a certain amount of flexibility and strength in your hips, knees and ankles, a dabble of core stability and a sprinkle of balance to top it all off. If you've never spent any time in this position, you may find dropping deep into a squat and staying there a little harder than you'd imagined, and you won't be alone. After all, our body adapts to whatever we expose it to the most, so if you've never hung out here before, don't be surprised if your body's a little resistant. However, if it felt a little clunky or 'wrong', a little painful, or you simply want to learn more about why you squat the way you do, then keep reading.

Strong Thighs Prolong Lives

It's no secret that our legs are important, or at least very useful, and I'm sure you'd agree that life would be difficult without them. The squat is considered a 'fundamental movement pattern' and is not only a great challenge to see how well those legs of yours work, but also a sensational exercise to *keep* them working. Squats can help with so much, from improving the strength, flexibility and balance of your legs, while also improving your heart's ability to support those two pins of yours.

I love my legs. I ooze with gratitude when I think about how much they do for me and how lost I would be without them. I have an incredible amount of admiration for the thousands of people who navigate life without them. My legs allow me so much agency in the world, to move freely at my command, and if you've ever picked up an injury that takes your legs temporarily out of commission, you'll appreciate suddenly how difficult life can become. Keeping those legs strong for as long as possible is a pretty good idea, and there's solid evidence to suggest that a strong set of legs lowers the risk of kicking the bucket prematurely.[1]

We all squat regularly, multiple times a day, usually without even noticing. Every time you sit down and stand up, you're doing a variation of a squat. There are many reasons why strong legs link with longevity, but I'm sure you can appreciate why the ability to squat helps keep us ticking, as the longer we can sit down and stand up by ourselves, the longer we can continue to move independently, and the more consistently we can challenge our heart to keep pumping all that bloody goodness around our body. This is without considering the impact that standing up, walking and general mobility has on our social life, which in turn has a monumental impact in protecting against loneliness, which works to both improve and maintain our mental wellbeing throughout all stages of our lives.[2]

The difference between squatting and sitting is that when your cheeks meet the chair, most of the demand on your muscles and joints is taken away by that squishy seat and shifted elsewhere, meaning they don't get the challenge they need to grow nice and strong. I'm not saying you have to sacrifice your chair and spend the rest of your life in a perpetual squat, but you want to make sure your body is strong across the whole movement, from top to bottom beyond the chair, in order to get the most out of your body's ability. Therefore, it's wise to spend a little more time squatting, and not just sitting. Next time you go to sit at your desk, why not sit deep into your squat for a while before getting comfy on your seat?

So How Should You Squat?

While I'm not too fussed about what your squat looks like, there is an 'optimal technique' for any movement you make, depending on what you're trying to achieve. For instance, say you're an Olympic weightlifter; you're going to need to move fast and powerfully to whip the weight above your head and catch it in a deep squat, so your squat strength and flexibility will be super important. So yes, technique is important for performance, but before we dive down that particular rabbit hole, unless you actually are an Olympic lifter, I'd argue that finding techniques that are comfy for you is more important than something that's 'most biomechanically efficient'. So, how do you do this?

Your personal positional preference will be determined by a few unique genetic components that make you *you*, as well as your current experience level. When it comes to your squat, there are a few main influencing factors over which you have zero control, but which I want you to know about before we start talking specifics. Two of the main contributing factors will be your individual joint structure and your bone length. Although we all, or at least most of us, have the same number of bones and the same types of joints, it may surprise you to know we're not all built exactly the same.

Take your hip joint, for example. Your hip is known as a ball and socket joint. This means your thigh bone has a big ball on the end of it which is supposed to sit nice and tightly into the socket of your pelvis. These bones are wrapped in layers of ligaments, tendons and other tissues, which connect to surrounding muscles, all working in unison to allow your hips to move the way they do. How this ball sits within the pelvis will depend on the structure of the surrounding bones, which in turn will impact your range of motion when squatting, walking, wiggling, or doing anything that involves your hips.

Genetic components such as your ethnic heritage can play a role in your bone structure. As an example, hip sockets among Chinese individuals tend to be shallower than the deeper sockets of Caucasian or African American hips.[3] The structure of our hips generally falls into one of three categories: anteverted, neutral and retroverted. Although it's not necessarily important for you to know which category you fall into, the takeaway is that not everyone is the same and it's important you find the technique that feels right for you, rather than looking for a one-size-fits-all.

For me personally, I find having my feet slightly wider than hip width apart, with toes turned slightly outwards, works best. You might feel comfiest with your feet hip width apart and toes facing forwards. I'd recommend starting with your feet hip width apart, toes forwards, and squat to see how it looks and feels. Then try moving your feet a bit wider and twisting your toes outwards slightly before repeating again until you find something that feels 'just right'. Try a variety of positions until you find the one that allows you to sink down low with the least discomfort or pain. If you've found squatting to be a little uncomfortable, playing with your squat set up can make a huge difference. I've found simple changes in foot position can have a drastic impact on how someone's squat feels, so go explore and find what feels best, or at least 'less bad' for you.

If you've played around and found a foot position that feels right, amazing work. You're one step closer to nailing your squat; now all you need is practice.

However, just because you've found one position that feels comfiest for you, it doesn't mean that is the only way you must squat from this day forth. Every now and again, practising with your feet in a variety of positions, differing the width between them and how far in or out you twist them can have plenty of benefits for developing resilient and robust joints across a wider spectrum of hip, knee and ankle positions, more capable of tolerating the randomness that comes with moving through life. As soon as you've found your confidence don't then feel you can't try anything else out; just don't go unnecessarily forcing yourself into painful positions. Remember, with every position there are things that feel good and things that feel less good. What this does give you is licence to politely tell anyone to mind their own business if they tell you you're squatting 'wrong' or that you 'must squat like this'. Be your own scientist and explore what feels good for you.

The second major influencing factor on your perfect squat is the length of your limbs. Here's a fun experiment: next time you meet somebody the same height as you, stand next to each other and compare where your hips are in relation to theirs. You'll probably find that although you're both the same height, the proportions of your body won't be the same at all. Some of us have longer legs, some have longer arms, some even have longer torsos. These differences mean we all move in slightly different ways, even when doing the same movement.

So how does this affect your squat?

Say hello to Barbara (aka Babs) and Wallace (aka Wallace). Despite these two delightful humans being the exact same height, Babs has a longer torso in relation to her thighs, in comparison to Wallace, whose thighs are conversely longer. This may seem like a relatively inconsequential difference in the grand scheme of life, and you would be right, it is. But when we start to look at how Babs and Wallace squat, these subtle differences become incredibly noticeable.

You'll see from Babs and Wallace that the ratio of thigh-to-torso length has a knock-on effect on how the squat looks. Those with shorter thighs will find it easier to sit more upright when they squat, while those with longer thighs may find it harder and need to lean their upper body forwards in order to stop themselves falling backwards. Neither position is better than the other, they're just *different* ways in which the body problem-solves unique to its proportions.

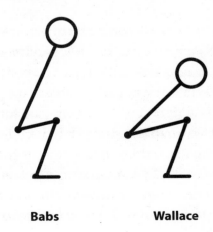

Babs   **Wallace**

Your body is an incredible problem-solving machine, and all of these unique adjustments are its attempt to keep your centre of gravity in the middle of your body to stop you falling flat on your face. In short, don't pay too much attention to how your squat looks, pay attention to how your squat *feels*.

My Heels Keep Coming off the Ground

This is one of the most common issues when trying to master your squat. As I mentioned earlier, in order to get low, you need to have a certain amount of mobility in your lower body, especially in your ankles. Without bendy ankles, the shins aren't able to get close enough to the toes. If you're unsure what I mean, lift your toes to your shins, and say hello to 'dorsiflexion', an unnecessarily complex word to describe your foot getting closer to your shin, an essential component of the squat.

Without enough dorsiflexion, the knees can't glide far enough forwards over the toes to allow your bum to sink down. This means either your heels will lift off the floor to compensate for your lack of bendiness in the ankles, or your bum will shift backwards.

To be clear, if your heels come off the floor when you squat, it's not necessarily a bad thing, nor is it bad for your knee to go over your toe, as long as it doesn't hurt. The body is supposed to move in lots of different ways and I encourage you to practise squatting in lots of different ways, too. In fact, squatting on your tip toes is a great way to build strength in your feet, while at the same time challenging your balance.

In saying all of this, I do want to mention why the flat-footed squat gets such good press. The squat is an amazing exercise for helping to build strength in your lower limbs. To be as strong as possible you need stability, which is important for maintaining balance. It would be harder to push you over if your feet were flat on the floor versus standing on your tippy toes, right? The same applies to your squat. I'll resist the urge to push you over, but I'd still like you to be able to get up and down with as much stability as possible. That way, if and when you decide to introduce extra weight to your squat with kettlebells, dumbbells, barbells or even a heavy backpack, you are in a much more stable position and you'll be able to lift more weight safely.

This image here is of a 'parallel squat', where your thighs are parallel with the ground.

This part of the squat is where ankle mobility (dorsiflexion) is challenged the most. So if you struggle to get to here, it's likely your ankles that are restricted. Conversely, if you can get this low but no further, it's likely that it's your hips holding you back. Keep practising your deep squat, but also check out the 90 90 (page 94), world's greatest stretch (page 104) and the couch stretch (page 114), all of which will help to unlock your hips and get deeper into your squat.

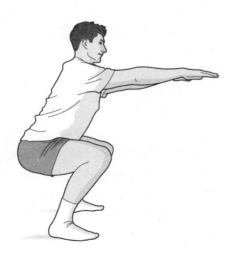

4 Simple Ways to Improve Ankle Mobility

1. Place something under your heels to raise them an inch or two off the ground. This will make it easier to get deeper into your squat without your heels coming off the floor, by artificially creating more dorsiflexion and allowing you to get your shins closer to your toes. If you've ever tried to squat in a pair of high heels, you'll know exactly what I mean. My preference is a small weight plate (1.25 or 2.5 kilograms), a thin plank of wood or a book – literally anything you can wedge under your heels that isn't going to wobble all over the shop when you stand on it. You can also buy 'squat wedges' online which are fantastic too. Over time, the more you practise being in the bottom of your squat, the more your body will adapt to being down there, gradually allowing you to use smaller objects and eventually remove heel props altogether.

2. Walking on an incline, like a steep hill or a treadmill, has been shown to improve ankle dorsiflexion.[4] Just 10 minutes walking at a 10-degree incline can make a huge difference, and could be a great pre-squat warm up. I'm not expecting you to carry a protractor around with you to measure 10 degrees, just whack it on a steep incline and get stomping.

3. Try kneeling down (as if you were asking to marry me) and then pushing your front knee forwards, over your toe, as far as you can with your heel on the ground. Do this until you start to feel a stretch in the back of your heel or calf, then hold that for 30 seconds on each leg before getting back into your squat. There's no need to hold any longer than 30 seconds, and repeating this

movement just a couple of times in between your squat practice will have a big impact if repeated regularly over time. You can also check out page 126 for the knee over toe split squat.

4. Spend more time squatting – practice makes progress!

I Can't Stop Falling Backwards

If you've tried all of the above but you can't stop yourself falling backwards, or your upper body falling forwards, try 'front loading' your squat by grabbing a weight and holding it in front of you. This is also known as a goblet squat (don't ask me why). You can use whatever you like that has a little bit of weight: a dumbbell, kettlebell, even a big bottle of water. This will act as a counterbalance and allow you to sit a little more upright without falling over so easily. If the idea of adding weight to your squat feels too intense, you can hold on to a door frame (or whatever's handy) and gain the same benefit.

Hopefully by now you're starting to piece together how you, as the unique little cookie you are, can wiggle into a comfy squat position so you can start to spend a little bit more time there, because remember: strong thighs prolong lives.

Now comes the hard part: consistent practice. Use the challenges as your guide. You may want to set time aside to do your squats every day, or be a little more spontaneous with your mobility snacks – either way, keeping it up is what really makes the difference. Don't be afraid to challenge yourself with a little extra weight if you feel comfortable with a bodyweight squat.

Let's have a little BREATHE, shall we? And while you're at it, have a shuffle and CHANGE PLACES.

Touch Your Tootsies:
Forward Fold

Ideal for: Hips,
Spine, Hamstrings, Glutes,
Spinal Erectors (Posterior Chain)

In this movement challenge we're going to explore the flexibility all along the back of the body. We will be looking at why touching your toes is beneficial for the body, and supplying you with tips and tricks to help you work your way up to reaching the floor with straight legs for the first time. There's going to be plenty of advice on how to strengthen your back and hamstrings, and for keen beans we'll look at how to go even further to get your palms flat on the floor.

I bet without me even asking, you already know how well acquainted you are with your toes, so the results here won't be a total shock. But I'm going to show you some cool tricks to instantly improve your flexibility, and to keep it improving week after week.

Before we begin, WHIP OUT YOUR CAMERA and film yourself.

CHALLENGE ONE: FORWARD FOLD TOE TOUCH

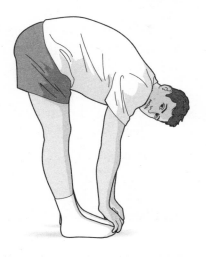

Standing, with feet hip width apart, fold forwards and reach down as far as you can towards the floor, taking note of how far along the front of your legs you can reach. When you can't reach any further, pause and breathe. As you exhale, reach a little bit more – this is your end point. This is your cold flexibility; we'll check your warm flexibility in a bit.

TAKE NOTE

- Rate the difficulty 1–10.
- How low can you go? Are you able to reach past your kneecaps, maybe halfway down your shins? Maybe all the way to the floor?
- Where do you feel the stretch? You should ideally feel it in the back of your legs and your lower back.
- Any issues? If so, where?

- Pay attention to how your body feels when you're in this position and note exactly where it feels tight or 'not quite right' – the more detail the merrier.

If you're sick of your estranged relationship with your toes and you're desperate to bridge this flexibility gap, then strap yourself in – it's toe touching time.

Why Do You Need to Touch Your Toes?

Touching your toes certainly isn't a prerequisite for living a fulfilling life or being a successful human. However, being able to fold forwards and pick things up from the floor without worrying that you'll get stuck there, and without the fear that one false move towards the floor will put your back out, has its benefits. Rather than it being a definitive standard, as always, I want to encourage you to explore what your ability – or inability – to touch your toes really tells us about your body.

In order to touch your toes by folding forwards, you need to have a certain amount of flexibility along the entire back of the body, from your heels all the way to your head. This section of the body is known as your 'posterior chain', if you want to get fancy about it. If you have any tightness along this chain, it'll make touching your toes difficult and you'll probably feel it. Although there's little direct evidence linking an inability to touch your toes with an increased risk of injuring your back, as a general rule of thumb, supple, flexible things are less likely to break. There is also evidence to suggest that if you've dealt with, or are dealing with back pain and feel fearful of moving in a particular way, the fear itself may make your pain worse.[1] Therefore, if you're a little nervous about folding forwards, gradually spending more time in this position with minimal, or at least tolerable discomfort may be helpful in building confidence and overcoming fear-induced avoidance of bending your back. Long story short: improving the flexibility of the back side of your body is never going to be a bad idea, and working on touching those toes is a great way of practising and enhancing your forward-folding bendiness.

Joseph Pilates (the inventor of Pilates) famously said that 'if your spine is inflexible and stiff at 30, you are old. If it is completely flexible at 60, you are young.' I know absolutely nothing about Pilates specifically, but I love the idea of shining a spotlight on spinal movement and associating age more with our ability to move than with how many times we've flown around the sun. I know this isn't literally how age works, but I believe that understanding the influence you can have on your body's ability to move in a youthful way is vital in helping to overcome our limiting beliefs about what we should and shouldn't be able to do as we get older.

CHALLENGE TWO: FLAT BACK TOE TOUCH

Touch your toes, but this time keep your back flat. Take note of where on your legs or the ground you're able to reach.

Rate the difficulty 1–10 and remember to take notes.

When you try to touch your toes while keeping your back flat, you take your upper body flexibility out of the equation, so this challenge acts as a much better indicator of how flexible the backs of your legs are, specifically the hamstrings (back of thighs) and calves (back of shins). This movement also reveals how well your pelvis can move, and whether it is able to tilt forwards, or 'anteriorly' (again, if you want to get fancy about it). If you flew through Challenge One and found caressing your toes to be an absolute breeze, but find it impossible to get anywhere near them the moment you flatten your back in this challenge, it may be an indication that you're more limited in your lower body, posterior flexibility. In this instance, it would suggest that more of your movement when folding to touch your toes in Challenge One is actually coming from your upper body rather than your lower body. While this isn't a bad thing in itself, it's good to understand the difference if you wish to improve your overall movement ability.

If you struggled with both challenges, then it may pay to work on improving the bendiness of the entire back side of your body. This is something we will explore with two spicy exercises known as the 'elephant walk', a movement that will help to mobilise the posterior chain, and the 'Jefferson curl', which will help to strengthen it while giving it a good ol' stretch.

If you found both challenges trouble-free, it's safe to say you're one bendy cookie along the posterior chain. However, as we know by now, bendiness is only one part of the movement equation, and we never neglect sister strength around here. So, alongside all of this flexibility, it's a good idea to learn how to strengthen the back side of our body to enhance our movement capabilities and build a more robust back side.

little trust with your central nervous system. You are slowly looking for the reassurance that it's okay to get a little deeper. Repeat this 15 times on each leg (30 in total). Don't worry if you can't comfortably do 15 on each side yet, just do as many as you can.

The more you practise this manoeuvre, the more comfortable you'll feel folding forwards. Over time, you want to strive to fold a little further forwards, moving your hands further down your legs towards your toes. When dabbling in any new realm of flexibility it's always a good idea to underdo it rather than overdo it in the beginning, so feel free to move at a glacial pace.

Once you've walked your elephant, stand up, take a few big, deep breaths and try to touch your toes again. Any difference? Say hello to your warm flexibility. If you managed to finally touch your toes after just one round, then congratulations. With regular practice you'll be able to do this without warming up first. If you're nowhere near your toes yet, don't worry, we're just getting started. For some of us, the change will take time to see, but that doesn't mean it's not all happening under the hood.

Take it Up a Notch: The Jefferson Curl

If you want to take your toe-touching to the next level, getting your palms flat to the floor and beyond, this is the move for you. It requires you to intentionally round your back, starting from your neck to your chin, rounding your shoulders and curling your spine forwards as you reach towards the ground, before reversing the movement and unfurling from bottom to top.

Starting with just your body weight, work up to at least 10 pain-free repetitions where you curl down to the floor, pause at the bottom for a few seconds, and hold that stretch (3–5 seconds

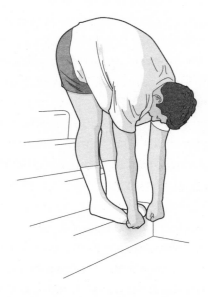

is great to begin with, building up over time) before coming back up.

As you gain confidence, you can start to add light weights in your hands (begin with 1–2 kilograms), and again work up to 10 pain-free controlled repetitions. Every week or so, if the movement feels good, you can gradually increase the weight by a couple of kilograms to slowly build strength in this bent over, flexed spine position. The additional weight will also help you deepen the stretch and increase the flexibility of your hamstrings (win win).

As you become bendier, you can challenge yourself to stand on a platform, such as a bench, to allow you to get even deeper into the stretch. Using a platform will make the weight fall lower than your feet, and over time will help you get your palms flat on the floor.

CHANGE PLACES. You know what to do.

Break the Internet: Hinge – Romanian Deadlift

Ideal for: Hips, Glutes, Hamstrings, Adductors, Spinal Erectors

Here we introduce another fundamental movement pattern: the hinge. If you're a gym enthusiast or you've experimented with weight training in your time, you've likely dabbled in some hinge movement patterns, such as deadlifts or Romanian deadlifts. These exercises focus on building strength down that posterior chain I keep mentioning (the back side of your body) by requiring you to 'hinge' at the hips.

CHALLENGE ONE: HINGE

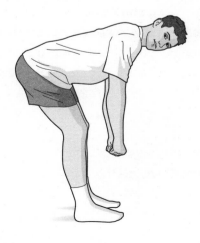

WHIP OUT YOUR CAMERA and get recording, it's time to hinge.

Imagine you have two pieces of wood, attached together with a hinge (like a door or cupboard). One piece of wood is your upper body, the other is your lower body, and the hinge is your hips. The idea is to create as much movement as you can from the hips, with relatively little movement from the rest of the body. Now, no matter how stiff you may feel, you're not a literal plank of wood, so some movement in the rest of the body is to be expected.

Stand up, feet hip width apart, toes facing forwards, and keep your knees nice and soft. If you're wondering what I mean by 'soft knees' – try not to lock them completely straight, but don't actively bend them; just think somewhere in the middle. Now you're set up in your stance, you want to send your hips *backwards*, as if you're sticking your bum out behind you, while keeping your upper body relatively straight and without your knees moving forwards. This is the hinge part of the movement. Imagine you have a rope tied around your hips that's pulling your butt backwards and that you're trying to make your bum cheeks (glutes) as big as possible. Keep pushing your hips backwards until you feel a stretch in the back of your thighs, or down the back of your legs (your hamstrings). When you feel the stretch, this is as far as you need to go. Pause for a few seconds before thrusting your hips forwards. Pow! You just completed your first proper hinge.

TAKE NOTE

- Rate the difficulty 1–10.
- How does the hinge feel?

- Which muscles do you feel working the most? Hamstrings? Back? Glutes?
- Any issues? If so, where?
- Pay attention to how your body feels when you're in this position and note exactly where it feels tight or 'not quite right' – the more detail the merrier.

This move, like many others, can be broken down into two simple parts. In this case we'll call these parts the hinge (when you stick your bum out backwards, known as an 'eccentric' movement, because our target muscles – in this case our hamstrings – get longer as you do the exercise) and the thrust (known as the 'concentric' movement, as our hamstrings get shorter). To get as much out of this movement as possible, we want to make sure the eccentric part of the movement is *slow and controlled* during the hinge, as this is where the hamstrings will be stretched the most, which is the aim of the game when it comes to improving our strength across greater flexibility. I move slowly, pushing my bum back, and count 1-2-3 until I feel that stretch. How long you hold it is up to you, but as the focus is to develop strength and flexibility in this position, a good aim is to spend at least 2–3 seconds down there, with the butt pushed back behind you, feeling a good ol' stretch before thrusting the hips forwards with some oomph (hence the pow!), then repeating it all over again. I want to encourage you to hang out and spend some time deep in the hinge, as this will really challenge the strength of your hamstrings in their fully stretched position.

To summarise: hinge slowly, feel the stretch, hold, a strong thrust forwards, and *voilà*, the hinge.

Performing this movement with just your bodyweight is a great place to start to play around and build an idea of how the technique can feel. Once you feel comfortable with the movement, you want to start adding some weight. Not only will this help build up some strength here, but adding load will help the flexibility gains too. If you're not quite ready to add weight, focus on holding the hinge, where you feel the stretch for up to 30 seconds. This will really help build strength and flexibility here.

What if I Can Feel It in My Lower Back But Not My Legs?

There could be a few reasons you feel sensation in your lower back rather than your legs, especially if your back is a little sensitive and you've never done this before. Feeling it in your back is not automatically a bad thing; this exercise uses all the muscles there, so it's normal to feel it working. If you've never put time into this move, it's logical that your lower back is going to start shouting 'Yo, what do you think you're doing?' As long as it doesn't hurt beyond tolerable levels of discomfort, we're all gravy, baby. That being said, you ideally want to feel this movement primarily in your hammys (hamstrings) and/or bum cheeks (glutes). So here are a few things you can do to distribute the force a little more to the cheeks and below, rather than just loading your lower back.

We need to make sure you're moving your hips backwards and using the muscles in the backs of your legs and not just folding forwards from your spine like the previous touch your toes challenge on page 71 (again, not a bad thing, just not what we're trying to achieve with this exercise). Have a watch back through the video you recorded and pay close attention to how your hips move. Do they move backwards? In other words, do you stick your butt out behind you, or are you just folding forward?

The simplest way to learn how to shift your hips backwards is to use a door. Start with the door open, just behind you, roughly a foot distance away from you, with your bum facing the open door. Attempt to push your hips backwards and gently close the door with your bum. Once you successfully manage that, move a little further away, an inch at a time, until you can't touch the door anymore, but you can feel the stretch down the backs of your legs.

If you have a loop resistance band, you can do a similar thing by tying it to a pole (or anything hip height that isn't going to go flying) and loop the band around your hips at the crease where you fold forwards. Walk out a few steps so that the band has some light tension and then repeat the steps for your hinge. The band and the door both provide external feedback to confirm you're moving your hips in the right direction. In turn, this should take a little bit of the load off your lower back and onto the cheeks and hammys.

Is It Bad to Round My Back?

If you've ever picked up something from the floor, you've likely rounded your back, so it's good to be prepared. However, when we focus on the hinge, we're trying to move from the hips as much as possible, which is why we limit movement in the back; this helps keep the focus on the glutes and hamstrings as much as possible. This is what makes the hinge different from the Jefferson curl in the previous challenge. No matter how hard you try to limit movement in your back, your spine will move when you hinge. There's no need to be paranoid about any and every movement of your back. It's impossible to maintain a totally neutral spine when hinging, so don't worry if you round your back a little now and again. If it does feel a little sensitive, it may just be that your body doesn't have the tolerance for this type of movement, *yet.* This is where starting with just your bodyweight, hinging as far as you can without pain and gradually building up to a 30-second hold will help build strength and confidence.

CHALLENGE TWO:
SINGLE LEG ROMANIAN DEADLIFT

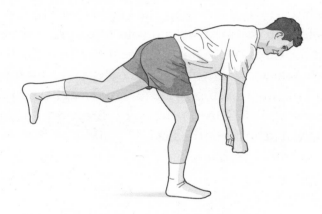

Say hello to one of my favourite exercises of *all time.* This single leg hinge variation is an incredible lower body stretch, and a strength and stability building masterpiece that will help you learn how to get your whole body working around your hips. There aren't many movements that tick as many boxes as this. So if you feel confident with the hinge, we're going to take it up a notch by lifting one foot off the floor. Ooh la la.

Starting on one foot, with soft knee (slightly bent, not locked straight), just like the hinge, focus on pushing your hips backwards, while lowering your chest towards the floor, using your other leg to counterbalance. Push your hips as far back as you can until you feel a stretch in the hamstring and bum cheek on the standing leg. Try to keep your hips square, with your belly button facing the ground throughout the movement. Pause when you feel the stretch and thrust forwards back to the top. Once you've had a couple of goes, try it on the other leg.

A great aim is to be able to complete 10 controlled reps on each side, hands free, without support!

Take note of how the single leg version feels and rate the difficulty 1–10.

If you struggle for balance, do this next to a wall or something you can hold on to for stability. Alternatively, place the toe of your back foot down as a stabliser; this is known as a 'kickstand' or 'B-stance' hinge.

You'll notice how challenging it is when you take one leg away, and that's what makes this exercise so special. The balance element requires coordination, and strength in your hips, core and legs, which all work together to stop you falling forwards. Next time you need to bend over to pick something off the floor, give this move a whirl. Once you feel confident and competent with this variation, don't be afraid to load it up and grab some extra weight while you perform the exercise to really challenge yourself.

The Key to Healthy Hips

If you're a desk-dwelling diva like me, spending most of your time curled over like a prawn, it's likely your cheeks and hamstrings will be neglected and rarely get a good stretch. Practising the hinge regularly is great for stretching the glutes and hammys, while the thrust provides a juicy bit of movement at our hips. When we sit down all the time in a constant flexed position at the hips, all the muscles around the hips get left behind, so they can always benefit from a good extension. Although this move isn't the only key to healthy hips, it's one of the most important pieces in our movement puzzle.

In other words, if you want healthy hips, don't neglect the hinge. And if growing an impressive set of cheeks is on your list, the hinge is a must.

Squeeze Your Cheeks:
Hip Thrust and Glute Bridge
Ideal for: Hips, Glutes, Hamstrings

I'm not talking about the cheeks on your face that your nan can't resist squeezing. No, today we're talking about your bum cheeks, your bunda, your glutes! Those big chunks of muscle on your back side are the largest muscles in your body, so of course we want to make sure they're nice and strong. If you've ever wanted to build an impressive set of cheeks, this exercise is key to your butt-building arsenal. Unlike the hinge in the previous challenge (page 79), which works our glutes while they're stretched, this move challenges them while they're squeezed, meaning the muscles are in a shortened position. Thus, strengthening the bunda across its full movement spectrum, leaving no glute-based stone unturned. No equipment is needed for this beauty, just a body and a floor to lie down on.

Before you WHIP OUT YOUR CAMERA and start rolling, let's test your cheek-squeezing abilities.

CHALLENGE ONE: SQUEEZE YOUR CHEEKS

Stand up and squeeze your butt cheeks as hard as you can. As weird as it sounds, I want you to give them a feel (you should probably wait until you're at home for this one, or at least do it on the sly like you're trying to rearrange a wedgie). Either way, give them a feel and notice them working.

If you're wondering why I'm asking you to touch your bum, it's because I want you to pay attention to the position of your hips when your butt is at its most 'squeezed' and tensed. If you struggle to 'activate' the glutes and feel your squeeze, imagine you're trying to 'tuck' your pelvis, pushing your hips forwards. Pretend you've got a £50 note held between your cheeks and someone is trying to steal it (just when you thought this challenge couldn't get any weirder). This position is known as a 'posterior pelvic tilt', and it will help get the best squeeze on your glutes for the exercise ahead, so remember this feeling and this position.

CHALLENGE TWO: GLUTE BRIDGE

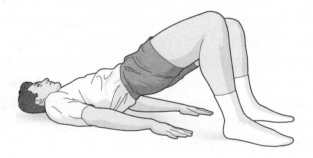

Lie on your back, face to the ceiling, with your hands by your sides, and feet roughly hip width apart. I want you to bend your knees and edge your feet (which remain in contact with the floor) up towards your bum. Ideally the bend in your knees will be at a 90-degree angle, and your feet will end up roughly a hand's distance away from your butt. From here, I want you to thrust your hips off the ground and up towards the ceiling, pushing through the heels. It may help to say 'pow!' as you do this move, though I can't make any promises.

Try not to think about lifting your hips as high as you can, but rather tuck your pelvis and squeeze your cheeks, like in the challenge above. You want to feel some serious tension in your glutes when you do this exercise. It's likely you'll feel it in your hamstrings too, and that's absolutely fine. As long as your butt is working, I'm happy. You'll likely find that the closer your feet are to your bum, the more you'll feel your quads on the tops of your thighs, whereas the further away your feet are rooted, the more you'll feel your hamstrings. If you can't quite feel your glutes working, play around with your foot position until it feels right for you.

Feel it in your lower back? This isn't a bad thing, especially if it's not causing you pain, but it's likely that you're arching as you lift your hips. Try to really focus on that pelvic tuck (posterior tilt) and this will help get the buttocks firing!

Once you're happy with your position, I want to see if you can do at least 20 reps with a big squeeze at the top and a pause for a couple of seconds before lowering slowly, in a controlled fashion, back down to the floor – this is one repetition.

TAKE NOTE

- Rate the difficulty 1–10.
- How does the movement feel?
- How many could you do in one go?
- Where do you feel the movement the most? Glutes? Back of legs? Front of legs? Back?
- Any issues? If so, where?
- Pay attention to how your body feels when you're in this position and note exactly where it feels tight or 'not quite right' – the more detail the merrier.

Found that a challenge?! Good! Keep practising. This is a phenomenal start point for boosting your bunda. It doesn't matter whether you managed 1 rep, 5 reps or 10 reps. Keep going until you can comfortably hit 20 before moving on to the next challenge.

If you found it a little too easy, breezing past 20 reps, and want to challenge yourself further, it's time to take one of those legs out of the equation.

CHALLENGE THREE: SINGLE LEG GLUTE BRIDGE

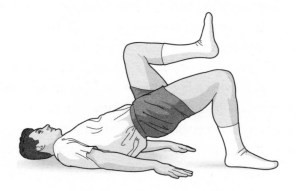

We're going one leg, baby! For this more advanced variation we're simply going to get into our glute bridge position and lift one leg in the air. Don't worry about how you hold your leg, just raise it in whichever way feels natural for you. This variation is an incredibly simple way of levelling up an exercise and challenging one leg at a time.

Once you're happy with your set up, see if you can manage 20 reps here too. Start with your weaker side, do as many as you can, then rest for 60 seconds and try the other side. If you're unsure which is your weaker side: imagine you're going to kick a football. Which foot would you instinctively kick with? This is likely your stronger one, so start with that leg in the air. If you have no idea which leg you'd kick a ball with, just choose whichever you fancy starting with the most.

Take note of how many you can do on your left and right side and rate the difficulty 1–10.

Why Should I Care About My Cheeks So Much?

Your glutes occupy a large amount of real estate on that body of yours, and having a healthy bunda is good for many reasons, besides the obvious aesthetic benefits. Your glutes are the literal centrepiece of your anatomy, helping to connect the upper parts of you to the lower parts of you, and covering the entire back side of your pelvis. These large slabs of muscle are broken down into three parts: the gluteus maximus (the main bit), gluteus medius (medium bit) and the gluteus minimus (the little bit), and they aren't just good to sit on. In fact, these muscles work to stabilise and move your hips in all kinds of ways. Without them it would be pretty hard to do anything that involved your legs, so, if you spend a lot of time standing up, it makes sense to make those buns strong. Conversely, if you spend a lot of time sitting down, it's likely your bum could benefit from an extra sprinkle of strength. Regardless of which position you spend most of your time in, a powerful set of cheeks will be an asset.

TAKING IT UP A NOTCH: THE HIP THRUST

To level up this exercise and increase the demands on your derrière, you can adapt the movement from the floor onto a couch, bench, or anything you can use to prop up your back,

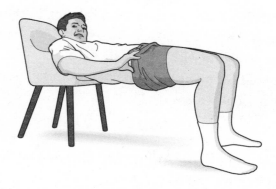

supporting you just below your shoulder blades. This change in orientation is going to help us work over a larger range of motion and challenge the cheeks a little more. This movement is known as a hip thrust and can be applied to the two-footed or single-legged variation. The best bit is that you can start to really work the buns by adding weight onto your hips with a barbell, dumbbell, a specifically designed machine, or even a backpack filled with things lying around the house. There are so many ways you can switch this move up, and I encourage you to explore! You don't need to master the floor-based variation of the exercise to progress to this; instead, have a play around with both and see which one gets your butt cheeks burning.

I Got 99 Problems But Hip Internal and External Rotation Ain't One: 90 90

Ideal for: Hips (External and Internal Rotation), Glutes, Piriformis, Psoas, Hip Flexors, Abductors, Adductors

When was the last time you gave your hips a good ol' twist? Welcome to one of my favourite moves for happy hips. For this delightful hip lubrication, you're going to need to get your bum on the floor, as though you're back in primary school (or kindergarten, for my American friends). Here, I'm going to introduce you to the wonderful world of external and internal rotation, two key functions of the hips, which get little direct attention in our modern world. Expect to feel a nice deep stretch as you challenge flexibility across the hips, explore your ability to twist it out, and learn some saucy exercises to help improve your current hip manoeuvrability.

But first, please WHIP OUT YOUR CAMERA, reunite your bum with the floor and we shall begin.

93

CHALLENGE ONE: THE 90 90 HOLD

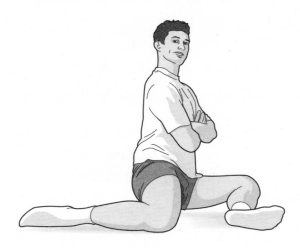

The challenge here is to see if you can hold this 90 90 position without your hands on the ground, while keeping your torso relatively upright, without falling to one side or being in excruciating pain? 'Good' will look different for everyone, but my challenge to you is to be able to sit into this position relatively comfortably for 30 seconds to one minute. I want you to be able to stay nice and relaxed, being able to breathe without feeling like your hips are going to burst! As always, there's nothing magical about these time frames; they're just a decent goalpost to show you have control of this position.

Once you're sat on the floor, I want you to attempt to make two 90-degree angles with your knees (hence the name 90 90). Sit on your bum with your knees bent and feet planted on the floor in front of you. Next, twist your knees to one side, like windscreen wipers, without moving your bum or feet, until your knees are as close to the floor as you can get them and resemble two 90-degree angles at the knee joint. Don't force it – we're not trying to rip your hips apart; we just want to feel a nice stretch! Once you've attempted one side, try the other.

Don't worry if your legs don't make an exact 90-degree angle, or if your feet or bum shuffle a little, or if you need to use your hands to support you to begin with. We're not here to obsess over trigonometry; the important part is to expose your hips to some saucy rotation. And don't worry if you find one of your butt cheeks has left the floor; that's typical of this position.

TAKE NOTE

- Rate the difficulty 1–10.
- How does it feel getting into this 90 90 position?
- How long did you last here?
- Can you get your knee all the way to the ground and keep it there?
- Can you keep your torso upright or do you find yourself falling over?
- Where did you feel the stretch?
- Did you notice a difference in flexibility between left and right side?
- Any issues? If so, where?
- Pay attention to how your body feels when you're in this position and note exactly where it feels tight or 'not quite right' – the more detail the merrier.

If you struggled to get into a 90 90 without your hands, don't worry! This external and internal rotation malarkey is a common area of restriction, especially if you've never flirted with this position before. A simple solution is to place your hands on the floor behind you for support. If this is still too uncomfortable, stick around and I'll show you how to adapt the movement to your current hip flexibility level.

If you sailed your way into the 90 90 position and held yourself upright without so much as a hint of a stretch around the hips, it looks like you have a wonderful base for hip external and internal rotation mobility – hooray!

What's So Great About the 90 90?

I don't need to remind you that when it comes to mobility, if you don't use it, you lose it. While that doesn't mean your leg will fall off if you stop walking, it does mean that if you want to keep a joint healthy and moving in an array of different directions, you need to expose it to as many movements as possible, as often as possible. Aside from the odd time I find myself tipsy and trying to do that Michael Jackson kick dance move, I can't think of many times when my hips are exposed to their full external and internal rotation potential, and I have a feeling you'll be the same.

This is where the 90 90 has a special place in my heart. While I can't promise it will help everyone, I personally found that working on my hip mobility had a huge positive impact while dealing with lower back pain in the past. I consistently found that during my worst flare-ups of pain, my hips felt tight as a drum. Regularly getting into the 90 90 position provided me with immediate relief, especially after long periods of walking or sitting down. While I can't confidently say my improvements came as a result of the 90 90 specifically, as the nature of back pain is so incredibly complex, nor back this with evidence other than personal experience, it makes sense to me that focusing on the quality of movement in the hips is likely to have a positive impact on the lower back. After all, they are neighbours, moving in tandem with every step you take.

I'm not claiming this as a 'magic bullet' for back pain, but if it helped me, it might help you. Or another hip mobility exercise might help you – I just want you to be your own scientist and play around. If you struggle with lower back pain or knee pain and you happen upon some restrictions and stiffness in your hips as you cycle through any of the movement challenges in the book, dedicate time to improve these areas of your hip mobility and you might just find it has a positive impact above and below. After all, we are one big chain.

The 90 90 isn't just about holding the position though, it's about developing the ability to rotate your hips, and this is how we're really going to help build some buttery hips! Challenge One looked at our cold flexibility. Now let's use this position to mobilise the hips and open up a bit of space before retesting with our warm flexibility. Introducing the 90 90 transitions . . .

CHALLENGE TWO: 90 90 TRANSITIONS

Sit down in the same 'cheek to carpet' position as in Challenge One, with knees bent and feet flat on the floor. I want you to swipe your knees down to the ground like windscreen wipers again. It's a lot easier to start with your hands on the floor for support, as the less upright your torso is, the less intense this will be on your hips. Please adjust as necessary until you're comfortable – we're not going for anything intense here, we just want to tickle those hips with a little stretch. Moving both legs at the same time, your aim is to maintain these rough 90-degree angles. When your knees touch the floor (or as close as they can)

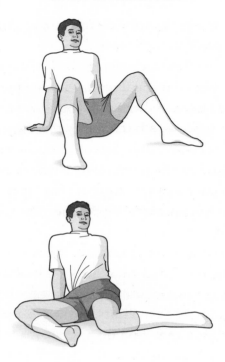

hold this position for a couple of seconds before taking your knees the other way, in true windscreen wiper fashion.

You may feel some clicking, clunking or popping in your joints, as you do this – that's to be expected. Our body is made up of so many different types of tissue, some hard, some soft and some made of goo. When we move these tissues will rub together and make noises that for the most part you shouldn't worry about, unless they cause severe pain. The pop sound you hear, like when someone cracks their knuckles, is just gas escaping your joint, sort of like a joint fart. This is why you can only crack your knuckles once, before you have to wait to do it again, as it takes time for the gas to build up again. These snaps, crackles and pops may feel good and provide a sense of relief from tension as we move into positions we don't spend much time in. The more regularly and consistently you explore these ranges of motion, the less likely you'll hear these pops and cracks.

If you feel some restriction in your hips while moving through the 90 90 transitions, make sure you move nice and slow and don't force your hips anywhere they don't want to go – just to the point where you feel the stretch is far enough.

To really get the juices flowing to your hips and loosen up the tissues around them, it's good to bust out a decent amount of these wiper moves, so I want you to repeat 15 swipes on each side before attempting to hold an upright position again.

CHALLENGE ONE (*RETEST*)

Now you've mobilised your hips and warmed up, let's retest the 90 90 hold and see if you notice any difference.

Take notes and rate the difficulty 1–10.

Notice any difference? You'll hopefully have found this position a little more comfortable with your warm flexibility. Using these transitions and holds regularly is a brilliant, low-impact way of moving your hips. But in case you couldn't quite get there, or found the transitions uncomfortable, let's look at some adaptations we can make to the 90 90 transitions to find a variation that suits you.

Your Hips Don't Lie

Remember the squat challenge, when we spoke about the individual differences in the genetic make-up of our hips? The same applies here. For some of you, attempting to find comfort in your 90 90 may be a doddle. Others might find it easier to get into internal rotation than you do to get into external rotation and vice versa. It might feel vastly different from one side to the other. All this might be due to the shape or even depth of your hip socket. If you feel a blocking or pinching sensation in your hips when trying any variation of the 90 90, don't try to force your legs into position. Our hips are as individual as we are, so it's far better to adapt the movement to avoid that blocking sensation.

Some Breezier Adaptations

Lean Back

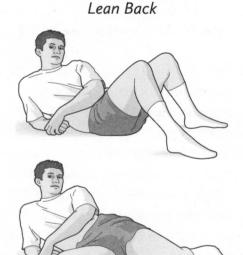

As I mentioned earlier, if you try to sit upright during the 90 90, there will be less space between your upper body and your hips, making movement harder. If you find sitting upright in this position too tough, place your hands behind you and lean back. The further back your hands are, the more space you'll give your hips to glide smoothly, without as much restriction. The feeling of a stretch like a delicious ache is good. A blocked or painful feeling is not good.

If leaning back on your hands is still too tough, you can take an even more chilled position all the way down on the floor, lying down on your back, propping yourself up with your elbow. You won't be able to rotate your hips as far in this lying down position, but if it allows you to more comfortably swish from side to side and feel a stretch without any pain, it's a win. Over time, as you become more mobile around the hips, you'll likely be able to sit more upright without as much discomfort.

Rise Up

If that still feels a little too niggly, a simple solution is to raise your butt from the ground so that your hips are higher than your knees. This might involve sitting on some yoga blocks, or simply the edge of a chair with your feet on the floor while you gently swish your legs side to side. This is a delightful way of adding a little hip TLC while you work away at your desk, when getting down to the floor isn't an option. Whatever you do, play around and find a variation that allows you to swipe your legs slowly from side to side and feel a good stretch, without any unnecessary pain. It doesn't matter which position works for you – it just matters that it works!

Can't Move Your Legs All the Way to the Ground?

If you can't get your knees all the way to the ground, don't panic; it doesn't mean anything's wrong. It will likely be due to either your bone structure (nothing much we can do there) or a lack of flexibility (which we can obviously look to improve over time). Either way, it's important to work with what you have, only pushing the movement to the point you feel the stretch. If your inability to pop your knees down is due to a bone restriction, you'll likely feel as though you're pushing against something solid like a wall, and you might not feel much of a stretch at all – maybe even a pinching sensation. There's little you can do about your bone structure, but it's still good to expose your body to these movements regularly; just don't try to force your hips where they're not supposed to go.

Where and When?

Finding things you do most days and associating a move with that thing is a great way of adding more movement into your life without it feeling overwhelming. For me, I slump on the sofa at some point throughout the day to watch TV or scroll through my phone. I've found getting on the floor and busting out a few rounds of 90 90 transitions and holds before I reunite with the comfort of my cushions is a great way of getting some necessary hip TLC into my life while still unwinding. Next time you slap the TV on, challenge yourself to get down to the floor and take those hips for a spin before you get too comfy. You'll be blown away by how the small, but regular practice amounts to amazing results.

And . . . Wiggle

When you're getting down with your 90 90, don't feel the need to hold it like a statue or move like a robot. Have a little *wiggle*. One of the best things you can do while spending time in any position is to give it a little jiggle and explore how the movement feels for you when you move about a bit. If you find a stiff bit, hold it there, take a few big breaths and relax into that stretch. Teach your brain that it's safe to be there. There are countless 90 90 variations worth checking out and exploring – this is just a starting point to introduce you to the movement and see how it feels for your hips. Discover what feels good for you and spend more time doing it.

The World's Greatest Stretch:
Spiderman Lunge Rotation

Ideal for: Hips, Lower Back,
Upper Back, Adductors, Hamstrings,
Glutes, Hip Flexors, Pecs, Obliques, Lats,
Rhomboids, Spinal Erectors

I didn't name this move, but I couldn't have crafted a more apt description if I'd tried. I hope you're ready to open up your body in all kinds of delicious ways (not as weird as it sounds; I'm just excited for you to feel the goodness).

You're going to need to get on all fours for this one (oi oi), so find enough space to lie down and spread your wings (arms). We're going to explore a few aspects of your hip flexibility with this move, specifically in your groin, as well as your bodyweight holding strength. Expect to feel a nice stretch across the front of the hips (the hip flexors) and a cheeky twist to limber up the mid-upper part of your spine (also known as the thoracic spine – pronounced like Jurassic, but with a 'th' rather than a 'ju' sound – in other words, the spine around your ribcage). This exercise is a sensational move for stretching almost your entire body in one go. So welcome to the world's greatest stretch (WGS).

Don't forget to WHIP OUT YOUR CAMERA.

CHALLENGE ONE:
GET INTO THE DEEP LUNGE POSITION

Once on all fours, on your hands and knees, lift your knees off the ground as if you're going into a push up position, but without the push up part. Once here, take one foot off the ground and bring it forwards, all the way to the outside of your hand on the same side of your body. This position is also known as a deep lunge, or a Spiderman lunge.

CHALLENGE TWO: DEEP LUNGE
REACH – ELBOW TO FLOOR

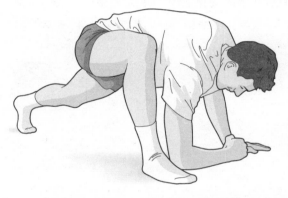

From here, take the hand closest to your foot off the ground and reach your elbow towards the floor to see how low you can get it, while keeping your shin upright at a 90-degree angle (without it falling forwards). Just do me a favour and take this nice and easy to begin with. This is your cold flexibility, remember, there's no need to rip your hips just to caress the floor with your elbow – you'll get there soon enough.

Go as far as you can until you can feel the stretch, BREATHE, and drop a little further. This is your end point.

Now do the same on the other side.

If you struggled to get into the deep lunge position, an easier way of wiggling into it is to start on one knee, as if you were going to propose, again. Then place your hands on the floor in front of you, so that your front foot is on the outside of the hand on the same side of the body, just wider than shoulder width, before lifting your back knee off the ground.

If when you get into your deep lunge you find it impossible to lift your knee off the ground, it likely means one of two things: 1) you need a touch more strength to be able to hold your body-weight in this position, or 2) you're a little tight across the front of your hip and down the front of your thigh (also known as your quad). We'll tackle this super common thigh tightness in our couch stretch movement challenge (page 114), but in the meantime, I just want you to keep your back knee on the ground.

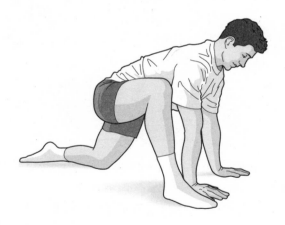

Now reach your elbow to the ground to see how far you can go. You may find you're not able to reach as far with your back knee on the ground – not to worry. This is just the reference point for where you are today, so you can look back and see how you've improved over time.

TAKE NOTE

- Rate the difficulty 1–10.
- How does it feel getting into this deep lunge position?
- Can you lift your back knee off the ground and hold yourself there?
- How close can you get your elbow to the ground?
- Can you keep your shin vertical, or does your knee push forwards as you reach to the ground?
- Where do you feel the stretch?
- Did you notice a difference between left and right side?
- Any issues? If so, where? Hips? Back? Wrists?
- Pay attention to how your body feels when you're in this position and note exactly where it feels tight or 'not quite right' – the more detail the merrier.

If your elbow grazed the floor with grace and ease, then congratulations, you're a deep lunge extraordinaire, and later in the chapter we'll show you how to take this movement to the next level and add it to your mobility portfolio. However, if you struggled with the movement, it's important to know that hope is not lost. It just means there's room for improvement and we're going to support that every step of the way.

Why is This Move Important?

On the surface, as you spread your legs into this deep lunge position and attempt to lower your elbow to the carpet, it may seem like a position with little transfer to day-to-day life. When we compare it to the likes of squats, balance or toe touching, which you perform almost every day, it might seem a tad irrelevant (although I'd love to see people regularly bust this move out in public on the bus or a supermarket). While you'll rarely need to break out a deep lunge to get you through your day, in part that's where the benefits lie. Daily life doesn't create opportunities for all the amazing ways our bodies can move, unless we create them. You may have more adventurous passions than me, but for most of us, our days consist of walking, standing and sitting, which often means that our legs only shuffle forwards and backwards while rarely getting a good stretch.

It's not just our hips that fail to explore their potential in everyday life; there are very few chances to get a little twist into our spines, or to move all the muscles in our back – and that's what makes this move so good. This stretch helps open us up in ways that not only feel incredible after a long day of stillness, but which also mean that we don't start to lose this range of motion. So, if you want to be able to get up from the floor with ease, roll around with your kid, grandkid, dog, cat, partner, or anyone else that deserves mild floor-based acrobatics, practising this move regularly will work wonders. The WGS helps you improve *and* maintain your ability to get up, get down and stay down, while hitting all the good spots left behind in life. And best of all? It will leave you feeling *really* good.

Now you've tested your cold flexibility, let's learn how to get the most out of this exercise by adding a fruity little twist. It's time to unlock your warm flexibility and see how low to the ground you can really get.

CHALLENGE THREE: A FRUITY LITTLE TWIST

Get back into your deep lunge position.

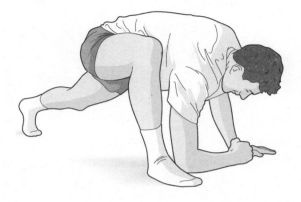

Take the hand closest to your front foot and lift it up towards the ceiling, then bring your arm as far behind you as you can, twisting it as much as you can. Push your chest out and imagine you're wringing out your spine like a wet tea towel. Take a big deep breath and, as you exhale, lower your arm and drop the same elbow back to the ground until you feel that stretch. Take another big deep breath, reaching a little further if you can. This upwards reach to the ceiling followed by elbow to the floor is one repetition. Using your breath is key to helping you unlock huge flexibility gains here, so make sure you breathe deep and relax into the stretch.

Like all the exercises in this book, there's no magic number of repetitions you need to do. I think a realistic aim is somewhere between 3 and 10 on each side, but the more important thing here is to focus on moving slowly and using your breath to move deeper into the stretch. Take your time. Instead of obsessing about numbers, think about how the movement feels and pay attention to where it feels stiffest. If something feels tight, hang out there for a bit longer, have a wiggle, and try your best not to get too tense. Chances are, if you focus solely on the number of repetitions you're doing, you're more likely to rush through them, so do as many as you like until it starts getting tough, then repeat that on both sides.

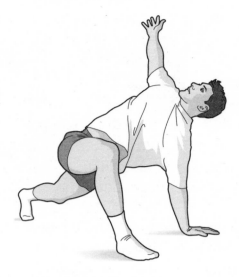

Take a 30-second break before doing the same on the other side – try your best to match the pace and number of reps.

Once you've warmed up both sides, you'll probably be getting a bit of a sweat on.

So it's time to retest your warm flexibility.

CHALLENGE TWO (*RETEST*)

Get back into your deep lunge position and retest Challenge Two. Notice any difference? You should find you're able to get your elbow closer to the ground now you're nice and warmed up.

Getting the Most Out of Movement

It's easy to feel as if there's a right or wrong way of performing these movements, but it's not as simple as that. As I mentioned at the beginning of this section, there isn't a 'pass or fail' mark for these challenges, and it doesn't matter whether you do them exactly as I describe or not. They're simply signposts, to see where you are in your movement ability journey. The most influential thing you can do for your mobility is move – *a lot* – and in *a lot* of different ways. This is where I want to give you full permission to play with this movement (and any in this book) and move your body in all kinds of ways. In other words, have a wiggle, have lots of wiggles. Set up in your deep lunge and move your hips side to side, rock your weight forwards and backwards, wave your arm in a circle. Do what feels good for *you*.

Quality of movement will come from regular practice, and learning what feels good for you will come from repetition, so do both of us a favour and don't get too hung up on performing any of these movements 'perfectly'. Focus instead on just doing them in the first place.

Common Issues

There are several common issues when attempting this position. If getting into any part of this position presented a challenge for you, don't give up yet. Below are some helpful adaptations.

Pain in Your Wrist?

Try clenching your fist and supporting yourself on your knuckles instead. Working on your wrist mobility will be really helpful for you, so I'd recommend checking out the push up (page 179), downward dog (page 153), tabletop (page 189), and hang (page 194) challenges to help build your wrist strength.

Too Intense on Your Hips, or Knee Hurts on the Floor?

Try putting your front foot on a chair, a stair or a bench. Raising your foot will reduce the intensity on your hips and also take the strain off your knee. Your hips will likely benefit from practising this, but also check out the 90 90 challenge (page 94), the couch stretch (page 114) and the front foot elevated split squat (page 127).

Desk-dwelling Diva Variety

I appreciate it's not always practical to roll around on the floor in the middle of the day. So, if you're screwed to your seat and still want to work a little groin action into your day, here's a bonus movement for you that you can do in your chair.

SEATED GOOD MORNING

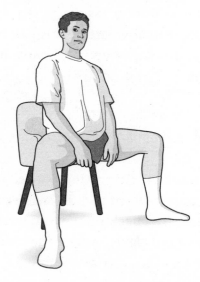

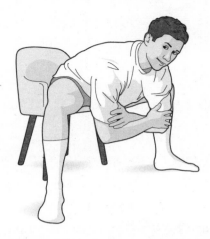

Scoot your butt to the edge of your seat and spread your legs as wide as you can, feet planted on the floor, knees bent. Keeping your back relatively flat, drop your chest to the floor. If you have a desk in front of you, you may need to shuffle your seat back or turn it 90 degrees so you don't headbutt your keyboard. Lower your chest between your legs slowly as far as you can until you feel a stretch in the groin, breathe, and lift your chest up. Repeat as many times as you like and, *voilà*, you've given your groin a good ol' stretch.

Over time, aim to get your chest lower down between your hips without much rounding of the back and minimal resistance from the groin. This is known as the 'seated good morning' and is a great way of improving the relationship between your back and your hips. If you have cranky hips, this is a great move to play with. If you're feeling particularly juicy don't forget to sprinkle in your fruity twist while you're down here by reaching one arm down to the floor and lifting the other towards the ceiling to get a little extra movement into your spine.

Hips Do Lie: Couch Stretch

Ideal for: Hips, Knees,
Hip Flexors, Quadriceps

As a stereotypical English person, I can't help but feel weird calling a couch a couch. To me, it will always be a settee or a sofa. Either way, you're going to need one of those cosy seating devices, something roughly below knee height to prop your back foot on, or a wall so that you can stretch down the front of your hip and thigh like never before. I'm warning you – if you're a desk-dwelling diva like me, or you just spend a lot of time sitting down, you're probably going to find yourself making a kind of 'wawaweewa' noise as this one hits the spot.

This is your nudge to WHIP OUT YOUR CAMERA and film yourself!

CHALLENGE ONE: THE COUCH STRETCH

Standing roughly a foot or two away from the edge of your couch, and facing away from the couch, lift one foot off the ground and place the *top* of your foot onto the sofa with the sole of your foot facing the ceiling. Lower yourself down so that the knee of the other leg is resting on the floor. If it feels uncomfortable on the bottom knee, pop a cushion underneath for a bit of padding.

The aim here is to get your bum close to the heel of the foot

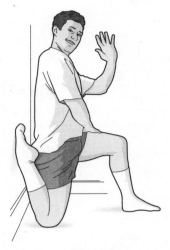

currently on the sofa, while keeping the torso as upright as possible, creating a straight line from your knee, up through the hip, shoulder and head.

Please note that this illustration was demonstrated on a wall, not a couch, don't worry if your foot doesn't look like mine. Using a wall adds an extra spicy stretch to the foot and shin, but isn't a prerequisite for this move.

How close can you get your heel to your bum cheek without your hips going backwards, and while keeping your knee, hip and shoulder in a straight line?

Remember that this is your cold flexibility attempt, so don't try to force it. Go to the point you feel the stretch, take a deep breath, and ease a little deeper in. This is your end point.

Now do the same on the other side.

Top tip: Remember the 'reciprocal inhibition' trick (page 75), where we tense one muscle so that the opposite one relaxes and allows us to get deeper into the stretch? This works here too: squeeze your butt cheeks (glutes) as you gently push your hips forwards and it'll help you get a little deeper. Just remember to BREATHE.

TAKE NOTE

- Rate the difficulty 1–10.
- Are you able to get into the couch stretch position?
- Can you get your back foot onto the sofa?
- Can you lift your torso upright?
- Are you able to get your heel to touch your bum cheek without your hips shifting backwards?
- Where do you feel the stretch? Your thigh, your hip, both? Anywhere else?
- Did you notice a difference between left and right side?
- Any issues? If so, where?
- Pay attention to how your body feels when you're in this position and note exactly where it feels tight or 'not quite right' – the more detail the merrier.

If the heel of your foot is lightly digging into your butt cheek while you maintain a glorious upright position with your hips pushed forwards and a straight line through knee, hip, chest and shoulders, then you my friend are a couch stretch connoisseur. If you couldn't quite crack the couch stretch position and it felt like the front of your thigh was about to rip in half whenever you tried to lift your torso upright, don't stress; I'm going to show you how to adjust the movement to make it a tad easier, then you can work on making progress over time.

Why Do We Need the Couch Stretch?

The couch stretch has been one of the most impactful stretches in relieving my historical hip tightness and discomfort, so I'm a little biased towards its majesty. While you should never rely solely on anyone's personal experience as an indicator of pending benefits and happiness, one thing most of us could benefit from is a little more hip extension, and that's exactly what the couch stretch does.

It's easy to spend the majority of the day with flexed hips, as we sit in a car or on a train to work, then sit at our desk before heading home to sit on our couch (it still sounds wrong). While this flexed hip sitting position isn't a bad thing in itself, when we spend too long in any one position, we neglect the movement needs of our body and the unused areas get a little stagnant. The large amount of time we spend in this flexed state means we neglect a well-needed function of our hips, namely extension. That's why the couch stretch and the variation below can be a sweet little addition to our lives, helping us to make things a bit more even-stevens.

If you rarely have a chance to extend your hips, you may have found getting into this upright couch stretch position to be impossible and felt the burn of a thousand suns up the front of

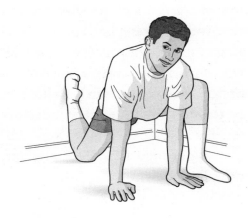

your thigh and hip. Please don't be put off by the difficulty. If anything, it means you've got a lot to look forward to from spending more time in this position. The main thing to remember is not to force it. You want to find that Goldilocks Zone of intensity, where you can feel the stretch, but it's not so intense that you can't take it. This may mean that you start with your torso leaned further forwards, and keep your hands on the floor, then gradually, over time, as your body starts to adjust to this position, you work on lifting yourself upright and pushing your hips forwards.

When Stretch Becomes Strength

It may surprise you to know that stretching isn't *just* about relaxing into a position to improve flexibility, this chilled out approach is known as 'passive stretching', hopefully for obvious reasons. While this passive approach is a phenomenal way of improving our range of motion, we must remember not to neglect sister strength when we have the opportunity to tend to her needs. This is where 'active stretching' comes into play and the couch stretch is a phenomenal position to play with and learn this active approach. The idea of active stretching is to get into the position where you feel the stretch and then actively engage the muscle you are stretching. For the couch stretch this means attempting to straighten your leg at the knee, by pushing your foot into the couch, as hard as you can, before relaxing back into a passive stretch. This allows us to get a little deeper into the stretch, but also to build strength in the muscles and joints by placing them under load while their fully stretched. This helps us develop control over our increasing flexibility, rather than just becoming a big floppy noodle.

What's the CRAC?

An example of how to use active stretching in practice is the 'CRAC' method, which stands for contract, relax, antagonist, contract. CRAC stretching begins by actively contracting the target muscle, in this case the quads along the thigh, by pushing our foot into the couch. A good aim here is to maintain the push hard for between 3–10 seconds, before relaxing, taking a breath and dipping deeper into the stretch, passively holding that position for another 15–20 seconds. You don't need to burst a blood vessel trying to move the couch with your foot, but you will need to exert some effort to reap the reward. After our passive hold, we want to contract the antagonist, the muscle on the opposite side of the body, in this case the glutes and the hamstrings, hard, for 3–10 seconds. You can do this by attempting to bring your heel as close to your bum by actively bending your knee as much as possible, while you push your hips forward and squeeze your bum cheek on that same side. Hold this contraction for 3–10 seconds. This is one cycle of CRAC stretching, which we ideally want to last for a total of around 30 seconds per stretch, before taking a little break for a minute and repeating 2–3 times. You can do more, but 2–3 rounds is a great start point to begin building some sensational strength in your stretch and can be applied to most stretches.

BONUS CHALLENGE: HIP FLEXOR LUNGE

When you keep your body upright in the couch stretch position, you'll likely feel the stretch more in your quad (along the front of your thigh). To squeeze as much juice out of this movement as

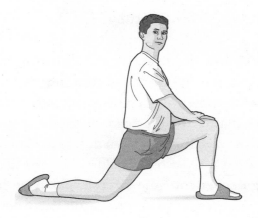

possible, you want to shift this stretch a bit higher towards the hip, too. I like to spend 30 seconds in the upright position, before thrusting my hips forwards (gently) until I feel a stretch a little higher, in front of my hip. Try to make sure you're not arching your lower back too much; while this isn't a bad thing in and of itself, you're trying to focus this stretch on the hips, not the back. To help you get it in the right place, concentrate on gently squeezing your buns (glutes). Spend another 30 seconds here and *voilà*. In this variation it's fine to keep your back leg on the ground if you don't have a sofa near you.

Fun fact! Your hip flexors are made up of five muscles in the front of the hip, responsible for flexing your hip (shock). One of them is actually a thigh (quadricep) muscle known as rectus femoris, while the other four are named the iliacus, psoas, pectineus and sartorius. There's literally zero reason for you to know that, but I think they all sound like Gladiators.

Spread 'em: Split Squat

Ideal for: Hips, Knees, Ankles, Quadriceps,
Hip Flexors, Glutes, Hamstrings, Calves

I'm not going to lie to you, this move is *sizzling hot*, and without
a doubt one of the toughest but also most rewarding of the
movement challenges in this book. This position aims to majorly
strengthen the muscles around your hips, such as your glutes,
hamstrings and quads, while getting a nice stretch on the hip
flexors, too. It will also challenge your balance and core stability
along the way. In short, a Bulgarian split squat (BGSS) is a single
leg squat that starts in the couch stretch position and requires
you to stand up then lower yourself back down to the original
position.

Don't forget to WHIP OUT YOUR CAMERA.

CHALLENGE ONE: SINGLE LEG STAND UP TEST
(BULGARIAN SPLIT SQUAT)

I'm not going to say too much about specific set up here; instead,
I want you to have a little play and see how you feel.

Start in a couch stretch position with your back foot propped
up on something just below knee height, then stand up. Now

lower yourself down, in as slow and controlled a manner as possible, back to your original couch stretch position.

You just attempted your first BGSS (also known as a rear foot elevated split squat for any enthusiasts out there). Now try it on the other side.

TAKE NOTE

- Rate the difficulty 1–10.
- Can you stand up from the couch stretch position?
- Lower yourself down too?
- On both legs?
- Which muscles do you feel working the most? Your thigh, your butt, both? Anywhere else?
- Did you notice a difference between left and right side?
- Any issues? If so, where?
- Pay attention to how your body feels when you're in this position and note exactly where it feels tight or 'not quite right' – the more detail the merrier.

Balance and core stability play a role here, so if you're worried about wobbling all over the place, grab hold of something for some reassurance and safety. You could place a hand on the wall, a chair, a broomstick – basically anything that will help maintain your balance while you push yourself up and lower yourself down. Over time, as you become more confident and stronger in this position, you can rely less on assistance and go hands free, baby. Or if you're feeling even more cocky, add some weights and off you go.

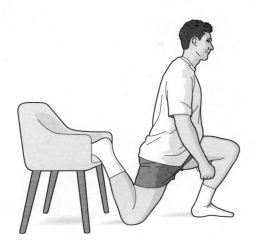

Feel free to mess around with your front and back foot place-ment to find a position that feels comfortable for you, and remember that you're not walking a tightrope, so you don't need to have your feet in line with each other. Your legs are like train tracks, so to help you balance, it may be useful to spread your legs to at least hip width apart.

As ever, there isn't a right or wrong way of performing this exercise. The important thing is that it feels comfortable (or at least not painful) for you. There is the opportunity to target dif-ferent muscles by slightly changing the position of your body, so it is worth using these modifications to help you get the best out of your movement. If you keep your upper body upright and your front foot closer to your body, you will work the thigh (quad) more. If you move your front foot a little further away and lean your upper body forwards, you will target your glutes and hamstrings. All of the muscles are involved in the movement, regardless of how you change your position, but if you want to shift the focus of the exercise to a particular part of your lower body, this is how.

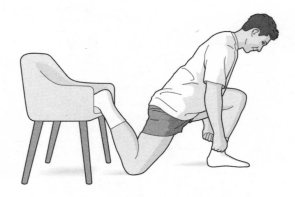

Similar to the squat challenge (page 55), the BGSS tests our lower body strength, which, as we know, is important for kicking it freely now and into the later stages of our life. The difference here is the focus on one leg at a time. Training one side of the body at a time is known as 'unilateral training', and it provides incredible benefits in minimising strength and flexibility discrepancies from side to side.

If you found this challenge too difficult, don't panic! This is a great target to aim for over time. In the meantime, I have two slightly easier variations for you to try (page 126).

If you passed the BGSS challenge – well done. That's another great sign you have decent strength and control in those pins of yours. However, if you really want to build strength in your legs (you do), challenge yourself to see how many you can do.

BONUS CHALLENGE: HOW MANY CAN YOU DO?

Complete as many Bulgarian split squats as you can on one leg. Rest for 2–3 minutes then try on the other leg.

How many did you manage on the left and on the right? Between 1 and 10 is a great start. Aim to build up to at least 10 on each leg before looking to add a little weight in your hands and challenge yourself further.

If you can manage more than 10 – well done. Now is the time to think about adding weights, such as dumbbells or a full backpack, to make it harder.

If you can manage more than 20, then you're a machine and I bet your heart is pounding out of your chest because that is one hell of a challenge. It's definitely time to add some weight to your BGSS.

Big Difference Between Left and Right

It's not a problem if you can't do the same number of reps on right and left. As we've discussed, we're all naturally asymmetrical to a degree. Most of us have a more dominant side of the brain and body, and a hand or foot we prefer to use. Our heart sits more to the left, our liver to the right. Our diaphragm, which helps us breathe, is higher on the right than the left. We all have unique quirks with how our skeleton sits (or stands). Some of us have one leg shorter than the other, some of our spines are curved more to the side. These asymmetries are simply part of being human, and luckily our body is incredible at adapting and working around them to allow us to move as one relatively well-functioning being.

However, it's probably a good idea to minimise any drastic differences in strength between limbs where possible, to help us function with a more balanced approach to movement. If you do find that one leg is much stronger than the other, it is worth noting which. Going forwards, it may help to start with your stronger leg, then match how many you can do with your weaker leg by taking breaks in between. Alternatively, you can always start with the weaker leg and not go so far with the stronger leg until the deficit in strength between limbs becomes a little smaller. Either way, you want to focus on getting both legs stronger.

Too Hard? Try These Adaptations

Knee Over Toe Split Squat

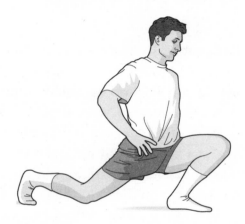

I wouldn't say that this variation is 'easier'; it's still a feisty feature in our movement challenge series. But it does throw the couch out of the equation, brings the back foot down to the ground, and focuses a little more on stretching the hip flexors and ankles, giving you another tool in the box.

Step forwards with one leg, with feet roughly hip width apart, so that one foot is in front of the other. Keep both feet facing forwards. This is your start position. If you feel a bit unsteady, do this between a door frame or next to a wall or chair for some extra support. Lower yourself towards the ground, keeping your back leg as straight as you can (it shouldn't touch the floor) while bending your front knee as far forwards over your toe as you can. Don't let your front knee drift out to the left or right; try to keep it in line with your foot. Go as far forwards with your front knee as you can, with the heel of your front foot on the ground and your back knee still off the floor. Hold for a big deep breath, then push yourself back up, using your front leg to drive you back to standing. Have a couple of tries, then swap onto the other leg.

Don't worry about how far you go, forwards or downwards, just find a position where you feel a stretch in the front of your hip on your back leg.

A split squat is very much like a lunge; the main difference is that your feet stay still in a split squat, rather than moving from point A to B and back. If you ever struggle to recall the difference, just remember the initials: split squat = stay still.

Front Foot Elevated Split Squat

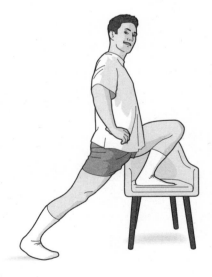

This movement stuff ain't about jumping in at the deep end, so if you found that too tough – maybe too tight on the hip or too painful on the knee – I'm not letting you give up on it just yet. Before you throw in the towel, we're going to make it a little easier . . .

All you need to do is raise your front foot onto something higher. The higher the foot, the easier, within reason. Raising your front foot up maybe one or two stairs, onto a chair or a bench, will make this movement a lot less intense on the knees, ankles and hips. Your job is to play around and find a height that works for you. A great ballpark to aim for is to be able to do 8–10 reps on each side comfortably at full range of motion, before inching your way a little closer to the ground. Sooner or later, with some slow and steady progress, you'll be working your way towards the more advanced variation, and I'll be screaming 'Look at you go!'

Whichever variation works best for you, stick at it. There is so much to be gained from practising this move.

Bounce, Baby, Bounce: Pogo

*Ideal for: Feet, Ankles,
Knees, Hips, Calves,
Hamstrings, Quadriceps,
Glutes, Core Muscles*

When was the last time you hopped, skipped or jumped? It feels like my youth was *filled* with jumping on and off anything and everything. It's hard to pinpoint exactly when, but one day, for no particular reason, all that joyful movement just . . . stopped. I'm not sure why we bounce less with age, but I'm determined to bring it back for the sake of your feet, and your entire lower body. In this challenge we're going to reconnect with our hopscotching history and revisit a fundamental human movement that often gets left behind as we age: the jump.

Before you panic about your creaky knees or angry ankles, this pulse-raising, calf-pumping, plyometric activity isn't a test of how high you can jump. Instead, it's about adding a literal spring in your step and bringing some bounce back into your life. For this challenge you don't need any equipment, however if you do have a skipping rope lying around, now is a good time to dig it out and dust it off . . . and don't forget to WHIP OUT YOUR CAMERA.

CHALLENGE ONE: POGOS

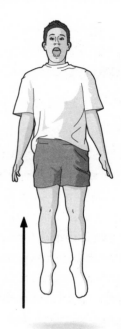

Stand with your feet roughly shoulder width apart (or closer, it doesn't matter too much, whatever feels comfy for you) and bounce on the spot for one minute, as if you're skipping but without the rope (or with a rope if you have one). Don't worry about how high or how fast, just *bounce*. This exercise is known as a pogo, for obvious reasons.

TAKE NOTE

- Rate the difficulty 1–10.
- How does it feel to bounce?
- How long did you manage?

- Any issues? If so, where?
- Pay attention to how your body feels when you're in this position and note exactly where it feels tight or 'not quite right' – the more detail the merrier.

It doesn't matter if you're just bouncing on your toes for now, with your feet in contact with the ground, or if you're hovering an inch off the ground with every jump. It's absolutely not about how high you can go; it's about jumping with a little joy, again and again. The aim here is to find a level of difficulty where you can feel your feet working and heart pumping, but without any unnecessary pain in your lower extremities.

Why Bounce?

Our feet carry most of us wherever we want to go. They're our daily touchpoint connecting us to the earth, but they're more than just two lumps of meat. If you've ever had any kind of issue with your feet, you will know that they are riddled with complexity. In fact, each foot contains over 26 bones, 33 joints, and more than 100 ligaments, tendons and muscles, all working together to help us bear our own weight and propel us forwards with a spring-like quality.[1] So it's a good idea to keep them strong, and bouncing is a great way to do that.

As you know by now, what you don't use you lose, so if you want to keep this bounceability in your feet, it's a good idea to practise a little. Thankfully, maintaining a spring in our step doesn't take all that much, just a bit of bouncing, hopping and jumping, known as plyometrics. This form of training involves explosive movements, where the muscles are stretched and then rapidly contracted to produce bouncy, explosive capabilities of your muscles. Plyometrics are something everyone could benefit from and they're easy to scale to your ability, simply by self-modulating how high you choose to bounce. Here are some ideas you can play with to progress your pogos.

Pogo Progressions

Once you can comfortably bounce for a minute non-stop, you can dip a toe in a variety of different pogo styles, starting with bouncing on your tip toes, to a full bounce with your whole foot leaving the floor. You can jump side to side, forwards and back, with one foot in front of the other. If you're feeling really jazzy, you can hop on one leg and throw in some side to sides, forwards and backs. Introducing variety to your bounce will challenge not just your feet, but your whole lower body, and its ability to absorb impact from the ground and produce enough force to help you bounce and keep that literal spring in your step.

How Often Should I Bounce?

The truth is, if you walk, run and are a generally active human, you probably don't need to pay a huge amount of attention to your bounce, unless you want to specifically improve your ability to jump, or develop your explosivity. That being said, if you're keen to keep your body moving and find it hard to squeeze as much activity into your life as you'd like, or else you don't spend much time on your feet, this is a lovely little activity to keep those feet springy and strong.

Although there's no set amount of bounce one can benefit from, I recommend putting aside a couple of minutes a couple of times a week to have a little bounce around your living room until you start to get tired. This will help keep the feet strong and improve the relationship and coordination between your ankles, knees and hips, which are all key for a mobile body. Plus these pogos will really get your heart working too – especially as you become more confident, comfortable and are able to bounce for longer!

To Shoe or Not to Shoe?

While we're on the topic of feet, it seems like a good time to touch on the rising promotion of 'barefoot' footwear, and the suggestion that other shoes are destroying your feet. More and more I see recommendations that we should revert to the ways of our ancestors, or at least attempt to minimise the support our footwear gives us when walking, running or generally going about our day. But is it really that simple? While some people report huge benefits from wearing minimalist, barefoot shoes, it's important to remember that one person's individual experience does not apply to everyone. Our feet are all different, and will respond differently. Rather than say barefoot = good and other shoes = bad, it's good to embrace the grey and say we don't know for sure. Some people will go their whole life without once considering the function of their footwear beyond how it looks, while for others it won't be so straightforward. Instead, when choosing your footwear, or lack of footwear, it's better to explore what feels comfortable for you,[2] and when it comes to training, if in doubt, it's a good idea to mix it up and expose your body to moving with and without shoes so you experience and are prepared for either.

Mixing Up the Bounce

There are so many ways you can bring a bit of bounce into your life, whether it's pogoing around your living room, adding plyometrics (jumping) into your gym sessions or, my personal favourite, skipping (or jumping rope). Throwing a rope into the mix is a sensational way of adding a skill element to the challenge, which I personally find less boring than just bouncing on the spot. So if you've ever thought about jumping some rope, this is your time. Don't worry if you're rubbish to begin with – we all are! Just remember that if you struggle with your coordination, you have more to gain from practising. Adding a rope brings some upper body movement to the party (and by now you know how I feel about extra movement), which works wonders for your shoulders. So, in this one exercise, you have an opportunity to train your feet, move your upper body, get your heart pumping, and improve your all-round coordination, which is incredibly good for improving brain function. Not bad, hey?

Stamina

One of the key components of mobility that we haven't touched on a huge amount yet is *stamina*. Having a strong heart that is capable of supplying the rest of the body with juice, and muscles that can carry you for long periods of time is everything. This won't be breaking news to you, I'm sure. Your heart is the engine that keeps everything going, and there's no point having all this movement ability if the main engine can't keep up. There's no doubt that most of these movement challenges and exercises will work wonders for the heart without you even having to think about it. The fact you are here, adding more movement into your life, means you're already doing incredible things for your heart. But, when it comes to a well-functioning ticker, it's good to introduce some sustained movement, for longer periods of time, to get that pulse up and keep it there.

Whether it's the classic walking, running, cycling, or any other type of cardio you can think of, if you move in any way for a sustained period of time, it's going to get your cardiovascular system firing on all cylinders. If I'm honest, I don't give a monkey's what your preferred method is; all I care about is that you're giving your heart what it needs. If, like me, you find conventional cardio a little boring, finding *something* that feels a little less mundane is a game changer. If you're lacking ideas, I absolutely recommend you give skipping a go, but if it doesn't work for you, all I ask is that you keep exploring. It may not feel like it, but there will be some kind of pulse-raising activity that you enjoy (or can at least tolerate). It doesn't have to be conventional; it doesn't have to look a certain way; it just has to tick the boxes for you. And in the meantime – bounce, baby, bounce, I promise your body will thank you for it.

Halfway Check-in

You're officially halfway through the movement challenges – well done for making it this far! Hopefully you're learning all kinds of things about your magical meat suit and feeling pretty chuffed at your body's ability to move in all kinds of wonderful ways. I'm also crossing my fingers that you've picked up a few tips and tricks for how to work these wiggles into your life, and I'm here to cheer you and your efforts along every step of the way.

But just in case things aren't feeling so fresh, and you've found some, a lot, or all of these movements to be really challenging, I wanted to check in to see how you're doing in both your body and brain, and to throw some encouragement your way.

As I've said, these challenges aren't 'tests' with a pass or fail mark. I get that's easy for me to say, and that it can feel pretty frustrating when you're telling your body to do something and it's just not complying. That is why I wanted to take this moment to explain why your ability to perform these movements isn't as important as the fact you're trying to do them in the first place.

All too often when we talk about mobility, we praise *how* we move rather than focusing on the most important aspect – the fact that you're moving at all. I want to make sure you're giving yourself the credit you deserve for getting this far, and for continuing to move your body, even when it feels tough, because when it comes to improving your mobility, the simple fact that you're moving more is *everything*, and I'm just really bloody proud of you.

Learning how to navigate and manoeuvre your body can be incredibly rewarding. Watching your own body's abilities change before your eyes is mesmerising, and there's nothing quite like those eureka moments when something finally clicks. But it can also be incredibly disheartening at times too, especially when progress isn't as quick as you had banked on. It might not feel like it now, but working through the difficulty, through the frustration, through the roadblocks . . . That is where the joy, the satisfaction and the spur to carry on lie. So, if it ain't quite clicking yet, don't give up. Keep going! And if you can't complete any of the challenges so far, that's okay – you're just where you are now, with all the improvement yet to come.

I'd love you to aim to embed these movements into your daily life and find joy in the process of improvement, rather than striving for an end result, because there really is no finish line when it comes to this health business. They're called challenges for a reason, so don't give yourself a hard time if you're struggling – it's perfectly normal! I promise they're worth pursuing. *Especially* the trickiest ones, because the greater the challenge, the greater the reward.

You're doing something amazing for yourself just by being here, reading this and moving your body more, and I need you to remember that the *only* way to improve is to move.

Keep going, you're doing great.

Your biggest fan,
Adam x

Core Galore: Side Plank

Ideal for: Spine, Hips, Shoulders,
Spinal Erectors, Abdominals (Obliques),
Quadratus Lumborum, Glutes, Adductors,
Abductors, Rotator Cuffs, Lats

Before we start, I'd like to address the dreaded word: 'plank'. Before you freak out and decide to skip this chapter, I *know* the plank is a horrible exercise. There are few things I like less in the world than holding the plank for any length of time. But I want to assure you that I'm not an absolute sadist out to unnecessarily inflict horror, nor would I encourage you to do anything unless I believed it was truly going to improve your life. This movement challenge may not be the most fun, but my God, it packs a positive mobility building punch.

Before we go any further, I want to reassure you that this isn't just any ordinary plank. No, no, no, this is a plank with a *fruity little twist*, which makes it a sensational movement for building a strong, robust body. The side plank targets strength and mobility around the spine and core muscles, and we squeeze even more juice out of the movement with some saucy side bends and holds. At the same time, we'll also be building stability in the shoulders and engaging the side of your butt and all around the groin – all good things. In fact, the side plank has so many positives, I think I'm going to have to call it the very best core exercise of all time. Sound any better? Hopefully I've at least persuaded you to give it a try.

The Side Plank Challenge Series

For this challenge, we're going to move through variations of a side plank movement, taking you from levels 1–6. Firstly, I'll show you the set up for the most basic version, before challenging your side-bending ability to help mobilise your spine and hips, and your ability to resist movement and help build strength in your core, from head to toe.

You'll be aiming to master two different side plank positions: the kneeling side plank and the full side plank. Both positions will help you to identify your current core strength and mobility abilities, from where we can begin to put together a roadmap to help you build a devilishly strong core and mobile spine going forwards.

This challenge is about zooming in on the robustness of the spine and its ability to move from side to side, as well as its ability to *resist* movement. Spinal health starts with our ability to move in a variety of ways *under control* – bending forwards (flex), backwards (extend), sideways, and rotating, are all of fundamental importance. But it also helps to develop the ability to resist movement, which is incredibly helpful for those times in your life when you find yourself carrying something heavy like shopping bags and want to remain upright. The side plank is a sensational move for introducing sideways bending and mobilising the spine, while working in tandem with the upper and lower body like the beautiful human chain you are.

As always, I'd like to preface this movement challenge by making it abundantly clear that your ability (or inability) to complete any of these levels doesn't make you any more or less of a successful human. However, a key component of movement ability is a strong body. Put simply, this is a bod that is able to move in all kinds of directions, but also able to resist movement when necessary. And this spicy series is a delightful . . . well, maybe not delightful, but certainly a *useful* tool to add to the mobility library. So, ahoy matey, it's time we walked the plank – the side plank, that is (sorry, I couldn't resist).

WHIP OUT YOUR CAMERA, it's action time.

The Kneeling Side Plank Set Up

You'll need some space on the floor for this bad boy, so get down on the ground with enough room to lay flat (see, I told you it wouldn't be that bad!). We'll start with the easier variation, the kneeling side plank, and then look at how we can level up this move and play around with a few more difficult iterations.

Choose a side and then lie down with your elbow on the floor to prop up your upper body. Your elbow should be placed directly beneath your shoulder and for this first level your legs should be bent at the knees with your feet behind you.

At this point, your hips will be on the floor. What you're going to do here is lift your hips upwards, off the ground, as high as you can. The idea is to make your body into a straight line from your knees to your head. When you get to the highest point you can reach with your hips, lower them back down to the floor. Simples.

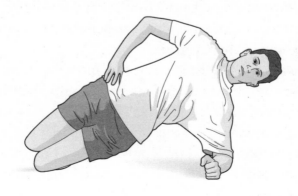

TAKE NOTE

- Remember to rate the difficulty of each level 1–10.
- Which level did you manage?
- How long/how many did you manage at that level?
- Where do you feel the movement challenges you most?
- How many did you manage?
- Any issues? If so, where?
- Pay attention to how your body feels when you're in this position and note exactly where it feels tight or 'not quite right' – the more detail the merrier.

CHALLENGE ONE:
10 KNEELING SIDE PLANK LIFTS PER SIDE

A good goal here is to try for around 10 controlled repetitions, but if you can do more than 10, don't let me hold you back. This lift is all about control. We want to move nice and slowly, ideally without wobbling round like a bowl full of jelly. If you're new to the side plank club, then jiggling about a bit is normal. Just keep practising and aim to reduce the wobbles over time as you build strength.

If you couldn't quite manage 10 smooth reps on both sides, keep going until you complete level one. If you nailed your 10 reps, it's time for level two . . .

CHALLENGE TWO:
30-SECOND KNEELING SIDE PLANK HOLDS

Here we introduce an isometric hold (isometric means *still* or *static* in the fitness world, because obviously we like to use unnecessarily complicated words to describe things. So, if you ever see the word 'isometric', you'll know to hold still like a statue). Again, this challenge is about *resisting* movement in order to test your core strength abilities. So, you're going to repeat the kneeling side plank lift, but instead of lowering down straight away, you're going to aim to hold the top position for 30 seconds on each side.

Set yourself up, set a timer and let the games begin.

If you couldn't quite reach 30 seconds on each side, stick at this level for now and build up to your hold on each side before attempting level three. If you've ticked this level off your list, it's time to progress to the full side plank lift.

CHALLENGE THREE: 10 FULL SIDE PLANK LIFTS

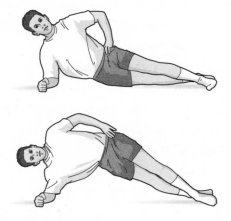

This 'full' version requires the same set up as your kneeling counterpart in challenges one and two, only with your legs stretched out straight, creating a totally straight line from head to toe. To help improve your stability here, instead of having your feet stacked one on top of the other, place your top leg in front of your bottom leg so that your feet are both in contact with the floor. From here, the only other contact point with the ground will be your elbow as you lift your hips as high off the ground as you can, before lowering them back to the ground: this is one repetition.

Your aim is to complete 10 reps, under control on each side. Not quite there yet? Keep practising. You've found your level. Master this before moving on to Challenge Four.

CHALLENGE FOUR: 30-SECOND HOLD, FULL SIDE PLANK

As in Challenge Two, the aim is to hold this full plank position with only your feet and elbow in contact with the ground, creating a straight line from head to toe for 30 seconds on each side.

You'll likely be feeling the challenge at this point. This exercise is meant to be tough – that's where the benefits are hidden. You may have noticed that not only is this exercise challenging for the core muscles around your stomach, but also your shoulders, hips, knees . . . your entire body, really. That's because this exercise challenges our body's ability to work as a chain to hold the hips in the air like a bridge (or more obviously, a plank).

Top tip: Focus on pulling your elbow towards your hip. This will help keep tension in a big muscle called the latissimus dorsi ('lats' for short), which starts under your arm pit and goes all across your back. This will help keep you stable.

Couldn't quite make 30 seconds on each side? You know what to do. Practise, practise, practise. Level five can wait; it's not going anywhere . . .

Smashed this level? It's about to get seriously spicy as you step into level five territory.

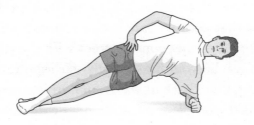

CHALLENGE FIVE:
THE SIDE PLANK MARCH (10 PER LEG)

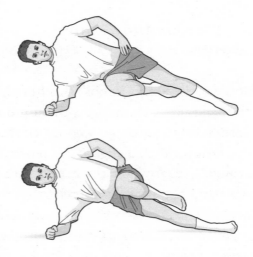

You can probably imagine from the title what this level is going to entail. Set up for the full side plank with a straight line head to toe with your elbow and feet supporting you in contact with the floor. Once your hips are in the air, in true plank fashion, march your feet. Lifting one leg off the ground at a time, bring your knee towards your chest in as slow and controlled a manner as possible, before returning that foot back to the ground and repeating the same with the other leg. I told you it was spicy.

This marching variation requires an extra element of core strength, engaging muscles on the inside and outside of the hips known as the adductors and abductors. Fun fact (kidding, it's not that fun, you know me by now): abduction and adduction are words used to describe movement towards and away from the centre of the body. Imagine standing up with a line drawn down the middle of your body, through your belly button. Any movement away from that line is abduction, anything towards is adduction. It always helped me to remember which is which by thinking about aliens abducting things and taking them away, and adding things together in maths.

Anyway, not only do these adductor and abductor muscles have to work hard, but your hip flexors also work as you lift your knees, increasing the demands on your shoulder and knee and adding one hell of a challenge to your core. In other words, this puppy ticks a lot of boxes needed for a strong and robust bod.

It's time to put that abduction ability to the test and give your leg a little lift with challenge number six.

CHALLENGE SIX: SIDE PLANK LEG LIFT

We don't have an illustration here, so for our grand finale in the Side Plank Challenge Series, you're going to need to use your imagination. Thankfully it won't take much, as all you'll need to do is set yourself up for a full side plank, then lift your hips in the air and lift your top leg as high as you can, as if you're trying to spread your legs as far apart as possible, like a side planking starfish (this is the abduction put into practice). Hopefully by now you understand the drill of building up to 10 repetitions and then challenging your ability to hold the top position for 30 seconds on each side.

This bonus challenge is really here to highlight that you can get creative and use movements as templates, adding some juicy extras that challenge different areas of the body. If you take this leg lift move for a spin, you'll no doubt feel one hell of a burn on the outside of your bum as you engage a muscle known as your gluteus medius. Abduction at our hips is one of the many movements left behind in modern life, which is a damn shame because leg spreading plays a role in healthy, stable hips. Although achieving this level of core stability may take time and lots of practice, it's absolutely a worthwhile pursuit towards that final goal of building a strong and robust body.

Don't be fooled by my six-level progression here; you don't have to follow them one at a time, but hopefully this will give you an idea of how you can progress and keep challenging yourself in different ways.

I discovered these side plank variations from Tom Morrison (@tom.morrison.training), someone I've learned an incredible amount from in the world of mobility and would absolutely recommend checking out. Pipped to be the 'greatest core exercise of all time' for good reason, they've become a staple in my core training ever since, and hopefully yours now, too.

The Fine Print: Asymmetry

It's likely that you have one side stronger than the other. This is normal and it isn't a problem that should worry you. But it's good to sprinkle some movements into our life that challenge both sides of our body – to help balance the books a little by reducing any wild differences in strength. The important thing is that both sides get stronger, not which one is stronger than the other.

BREATHE. A sigh of sweet relief, you survived the plank.

Around the World:
Shoulder Dislocates

Ideal for: Shoulders,
Rotator Cuffs, Chest, Arms

While the name of this challenge might be a little scary, I *promise* there'll be no shoulders popping out of sockets around here (at least I hope not). Instead, I welcome you to one of my first ports of call for anyone dealing with a little shoulder discomfort. Once you take it for a whirl, you'll see how simple and effective it can be for helping to stretch and lube up your shoulders, keeping them strong, healthy and ready for anything. Well, almost anything.

For this challenge you'll need a resistance band or towel. My personal preference is a resistance band as it allows some extra adjustment based on your flexibility level, but if you don't have access to one, a towel will do just fine.

CHALLENGE: HOW CLOSE ARE YOUR HANDS?

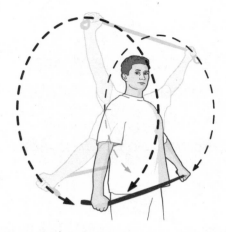

A shoulder 'dislocate' in this context involves holding your prop with both hands, in front of your body with palms facing down. The aim is to lift the band or whichever piece of equipment you've found around the house up above your head, and then all the way behind you in one large circular motion, until you reach your back or bum. The catch is, you have to keep your arms straight the *whole* time. The further apart your hands, the easier the movement will be; the closer they are, the bigger the challenge. Once you've gone as far as you can behind you, reverse the movement and slowly bring your arms all the way back to where they started in front of you. *Voilà* – the shoulder dislocate. Wasn't so scary after all, huh?

If you have to bend your arms, your hands are too close together. Move them further apart and identify how wide along the band, towel (or whatever you use) your hands should be in order to make the full dislocate shoulder motion.

Once you've found your zone, it can help to mark it with a pen or some tape to track where you started and see how you improve over time – just like my nan used to do with my height on the wall, only less cute.

TAKE NOTE

- Rate the difficulty 1–10.
- Can you manage a full circle from front to back without bending your arms?
- Where do you feel the stretch the most?
- How close / far apart are your hands?
- Any issues at any point during the movement? If so, where?
- Pay attention to how your body feels when you're in this position and note exactly where it feels tight or 'not quite right' – the more detail the merrier.

Truth be told, this challenge is less about 'how close can you get your hands together' and more about finding a hand distance that's comfortable for you, where you can still feel a good stretch across your shoulders, chest and arms. While most of us don't need turbo flex in our shoulders to live a good life, possessing shoulders that can move nice and smoothly will *always* be a good thing. By now I'm sure you appreciate that a strong and bendy joint is often a healthy one, so it's important to work on developing the ability to move any joint along all its possible lines of direction, with control under resistance. These shoulder dislocates are a cheeky way of doing just that: keeping your shoulders greased, grooved and oiled up with just a few simple bits of equipment, this is one effective way for us to give our rotator cuff muscles some much-needed TLC.

What the Cuff?

You may or may not have heard of the fairly notorious group of muscles known as the 'rotator cuff'. The cuff actually refers to four different muscles: the supraspinatus, infraspinatus, subscapularis and teres minor. You really do not need to remember these names, and I imagine that's why they lumped them all together and gave them the much more memorable name 'rotator cuff'. All you really need to take away from this anatomy mumbo jumbo is that it's a group of muscles that helps rotate and maintain stability within the shoulder, and that it's a good idea to keep them moving, with strength and bendiness in mind. Though do keep in mind that if you're new to this movement, go gently and don't try to force anything.

Although healthy shoulders 'should' be able to perform this movement, if you've dealt with a shoulder injury in the past, it can be incredibly tough to begin with. Stay within your pain-free range of motion, even if that means not going all the way around. Don't go too hard – a light stretch is more than enough for now. You'll find that exposing your shoulders to a regular gentle stretch will allow the cuff to start to relax and move further in this circular motion over time.

A resistance band is great for this exercise. The elastic of the band adds an element of 'flexibility' and allows your shoulders and hands to adjust their position to suit your body. If you don't have access to one, they are relatively cheap and can be bought for around a tenner. I recommend the 'loop resistance bands', but don't worry too much about that. As long as it's a band, has some resistance and it's in your price range, it'll do the job. Whatever you use, make sure you give it a go and do not let any initial 'ooowwee' kind of feeling put you off. Just open your hands out a little further and give it another spin.

Beyond the Shoulders . . .

This might be a shoulder dislocate, but the benefits go way beyond that. Often when we talk about movement in the body, we refer to it in isolated terms, pinpointing the *shoulders*, or the *arms*, or the *feet*. But as humans we rarely move in true isolation, and most of the time when we shift one bit, we move something next door to it too (remember the analogy of the spine being like one big chain, for example). You'll likely have felt this in practice during the dislocate, as you lifted your arms in front of you, waved them over your head and started to reach and drop them behind you in a big sort of Y shape.

As well as one hell of a stretch in your shoulders, you'll also have mobilised the next-door neighbours – the chest, as well as the arms and into the biceps. Our shoulders work in tandem with all of the musculature in our upper body, and when we wave our arms in this circular fashion, it engages all the connecting tissues too, stretching and challenging them in ways they're not used to in day-to-day life. If you're a professional prawn (aka desk-dwelling diva) like me, it's a good idea to find ways of stretching and opening up your chest with what's known as thoracic extension (or as I like to call it, the anti-prawn). If you're unsure what I mean by this, puff your chest out: this is thoracic extension. These dislocates are killer for making sure our body is getting the upper body movement variety it needs, and offers a great antidote if you've spent too long in any one position.

If you're looking to take the intensity down a touch, you don't have to be standing – you can sit or kneel too, and as always, I want to encourage you to have a wiggle throughout this movement. You don't have to *just* go forwards and back above your head, you have licence to whirl your arms however you please. Try moving one arm at a time or bending side to side as you explore your shoulders' wonderful movement capabilities, while becoming best friends with the dislocate and all its vibrant variations.

Putting it into Practice

Like all of these movement challenges, I want to encourage you to find ways to fit this movement into your daily life beyond the limits of dedicated exercise sessions. This could mean taking your resistance band to work so you have it on hand (I know it might look weird, but you never know, you might inspire a co-worker), storing it next to your desk at home, or taking your towel for a spin before and after you shower. Whatever you do, the best results will always come from squeezing this mega stretch in daily, or as often as possible.

The Double D: Downward Dog

Ideal for: Shoulders, Scapulas,
Wrists, Hips, Knees

For all my Yogi bears in the crowd, it's time to introduce this canine classic, which is an absolute banger when it comes to building overhead shoulder strength and stability, while also strengthening the forearms and wrists. As an added bonus, there's also a tasty stretch down the back of the legs, too.

I know many of you will already be familiar with this position, but in case you've never got down with the dog, I want to help you unlock all the goodness of this move and remind you that you don't have to be a yoga enthusiast to benefit from some of its positions. All you need to get started with this barkingly brilliant move, is enough space on the floor to lie down and some mild enthusiasm.

Before we dabble in the dog, let's take your overhead shoulder mobility for a spin, just make sure you WHIP OUT YOUR CAMERA and get recording.

CHALLENGE ONE: OVERHEAD MOBILITY

Stand up, with your arms by your side, then lift your arms above your head in a straight line without curving your lower back.

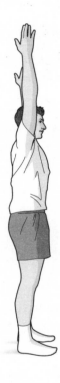

This is a really simple challenge to see how well you can move your shoulders overhead. If you struggle to get them up without arching your lower back, it's likely you have a little restriction in your overhead mobility, which may be due to tightness in your lats down the side of your back or in your upper and mid-back (remember that thoracic part of your spine that sounds like Jurassic but has nothing to do with dinosaurs? That!). This exercise is going to help you open up that upper back of yours and get your shoulders motoring like never before.

Without further ado, let's move on to the downward dog. Woof.

CHALLENGE TWO: DO THE DOG

All I want you to do for this challenge is lift yourself into the downward dog position and see how long you can hold it and how deep you can go. So exactly how do you do that, you ask?

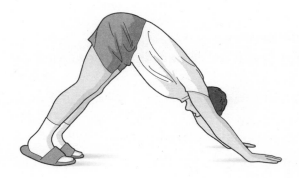

Start by getting yourself down to the floor in a high press up position with straight arms. With both hands on the floor, roughly shoulder width apart, legs straight, feet hip width apart with toes pressed to the ground, you're going to lift your bum in the air as high as you can. Keeping your legs as straight as you can, think about pushing the floor away from you, drop your chest and bring your head down between your arms, aiming to create straight lines from your hands to your hips and your hips to your feet, like two sides of a triangle. Depending on the flexibility of the backs of your legs, your feet will either be on tip toes or fully touching the ground in a flat position. Don't worry too much about what yours are doing right now, just find what's comfortable for you and focus on creating two straight lines with your upper and lower body.

If you're wondering what I mean by getting 'deep into the dog', what we want to see is a fairly pointed, deeply folded forwards shape during this move, almost like an arrow with your bum being the tip.

Remember this is your cold flexibility. Don't force it. Just dabble and see how it feels. We'll warm up and retest soon enough!

TAKE NOTE

- Rate the difficulty 1–10.
- How does it feel getting into this downward dog position?
- Can you lift your bum to the sky and hold yourself there? If so, for how long?
- Can you straighten your legs?
- Can you get your feet flat or are you up on your toes?
- Can you make a straight line from hands to hips?
- Any issues? If so, where?
- Pay attention to how your body feels when you're in this position and note exactly where it feels tight or 'not quite right' – the more detail the merrier.

If you're a downward dogging don and well versed in this move, you'll likely breeze through this set up. If you're new to the dog pack, this movement can feel a little sticky. As always, we'll play with some alternative set ups, but first: why should we bother getting down with the dog at all?

Why Do the Downward Dog?

Not only does this move have a great name, but for such a relatively simple position, you are going to get some mega benefits. Getting down with the dog requires a certain amount of strength and flexibility in our shoulders, especially in an overhead position. Come to think about it, when was the last time you put your arms above your head? Probably not enough! The shoulder is the most mobile joint in the body (when working properly). It is a ball and socket joint (just like your hips), but your shoulder joint is much shallower and relies on your shoulder blade (also known as the scapula) working together to help you wave your arms in the air like you just don't care. As it's the most mobile joint in the body, it is super helpful to build stability here, and that's exactly what this exercise does. You may notice when playing with this downward dog that you feel an incredible stretch, and maybe some pops and cracks in your upper back and around your ribcage. Remember, this is all good and just a sign of gas escaping from your joints.

Not only does this move work the shoulders and shoulder blades, but you may also have noticed it requires a level of 'forward folding' (hip flexion) and flexibility down the back of your body (remember our posterior chain!). The sensation may feel similar to touching your toes, just less extreme, which makes this a nice 'two birds with one stone' sort of move. To really pop a cherry on top, the downward dog also helps us introduce some weight-bearing into our hands, wrists and forearms, stimulates all those core muscles, and gives the calves a good ol' stretch. In other words, it's sensational.

To maximise that juicy calf stretch (the back of your lower leg), while you've got your bum in the air, in full DD mode, stretch your heels down to the floor, either together or one foot at a time.

The plan is to get your feet as flat as possible on the floor. The further away your hands are from your legs, the harder it will be to get your feet flat, so don't worry if you can't manage it. The aim of this game is just to feel this super stretch. Feel free to gently pulse each heel down to the ground to get those movement juices flowing before holding in position.

Whether you're looking to build a more robust body overall, or specifically sculpting stable shoulders so you can carry things above your head with pride, pick things off the top shelf with ease, or support yourself more safely should you fall, the downward facing dog is worth practising.

Too Tricky? Try This!

If you find jumping straight into the DD too tough on the body, a simple tweak to make it more accessible is to start with your hands on a wall or a chair rather than on the floor. Stand just further than arm's length away from the wall, reach out and place your palms on the surface, then drop your chest to face the floor while keeping your legs as straight as possible. We'll call this the

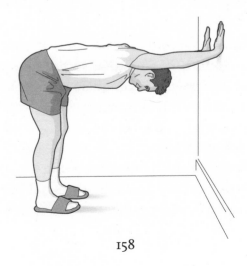

wall dog (I don't think it's actually called that, but it has a nice ring to it). This is a great way of taking pressure from your hands and shoulders while still exposing your body to a similar movement. Over time, you can progress the move by shifting your hands further down the wall, and your feet further away. When you feel like you've mastered the wall, try moving your hands down onto a sofa, a step, and eventually you might even make it down to the ground as you get more confident.

If the DD feels fine on the shoulders but you can't for the life of you keep your legs straight, don't let it deter you. Keep your knees bent and practise what you can do. If this is you, I'd recommend spending time improving your touch your toes (page 71), hinge (page 79) and world's greatest stretch (page 104) challenges.

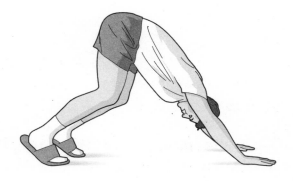

Time to Mobilise

As always, we want to mobilise and get deeper into the position by lengthening all those involved body parts and retesting our warm flexibility to strengthen that new range of motion.

To do this we're simply going to transition from a high push up position into our downward dog, hold for a few seconds, and then back to the push up (don't worry, I'm not actually going to make you do any push ups). Make sure you're moving nice and slow from point A to B. This dog likes control and authority, not to be rushed. This is going to help build strength across the whole range of motion, while also getting that body of yours nice and warm. Once you've completed roughly 10–15 controlled repetitions, or as many as you can, take a 30-second to 1-minute breather and retest your flexibility from Challenge Two.

CHALLENGE TWO (*RETEST*)

Hopefully you're at least marginally deeper into the dog and feeling a nice stretch across your upper back, the front of your ribcage and down the backs of your legs.

Now it's time to supercharge this shoulder-stabilising exercise with a little bonus challenge.

BONUS CHALLENGE: ONE HAND TOE TAPPER

If you're feeling confident with your downward dog and want to learn how to take it up a notch, get back into position. This time, when you stick your bum in the air and fold your chest towards your legs, I want you to lift one hand from the ground, reach that hand backwards to the *opposite* foot with as much control as you can, before placing it back where it started. This spicy twist of events requires your solo shoulder to do the brunt of the work to stabilise your body. Once you've reached one hand to one toe, try with the other side.

You may find one shoulder feels a lot stronger than the other, and if that's the case, spending a little more time focusing on the weaker side would be sensible. If you struggle to keep control with just one hand, focus on nailing your DD transitions and holds with as much control as possible and you'll be mastering the one hand toe tapper in no time.

To get the most out of this exercise it's good to play around with both the transitions and the holds. Work towards feeling more confident and comfortable, bouncing slowly between these positions and holding any from point A (your pre-push up position) to point B (full-blown downward dog). Never be afraid to have a wiggle along the way if you feel a little stiff, and if it feels nice, do it twice or thrice for all I care, as long as you're moving, I'm a happy pup.

I'm a Snake: The Cobra

Ideal for: Lower Back, Abdominals, Wrists, Hands

Now, we ain't talking about those feisty legless fellas with the big neck that like to hiss and spit at things. We're talking about another yoga classic: the cobra (I personally really enjoy how many of these moves are named after animals).

This slithery floor-based move introduces some much-needed spinal extension into our lives, specifically in the lower back area known as the lumbar spine. This beautifully simple move just needs a floor and enough space to lay stretched out on your belly.

Don't forget to WHIP OUT YOUR CAMERA!

CHALLENGE ONE: THE COBRA

Lie face down, legs straight, with toes pointed, like a ballerina. Place your hands on the floor by the side of your ribs and push your upper body off the ground until your arms are straight, or as straight as you can get them. The crown of your head should point to the ceiling with your chest facing to the front. Your hip should stay in contact with the ground, creating a big curve in your back. Pull your shoulder blades back and down, squeeze your bum cheeks, take a big, deep breath and sigh it all out, ahhhh. Relax and hold that position for a few deep breaths, *et voilà*, you have *le cobra*.

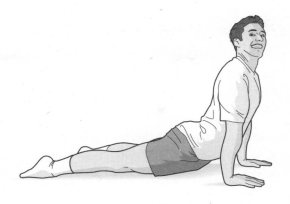

As always, I want to encourage you to play around with your cobra set up and find what feels best for you. The main focus of this move is to feel a nice stretch across your abs and down the front of your torso. You'll likely feel your lower back working here too, but if you find it too difficult to lift yourself upright, don't be afraid to start on your elbows or shimmy your hand position. Of course, you can simply not push yourself so high. Remember this is your cold flexibility, so don't force it, just go to the point you feel the stretch, take a big breath, and lower your chest to the floor again. To test your warm flexibility, I want you to repeat this 10 times, with a breath at the top of each cobra. This is known as a cobra push up and is a great way of getting a little movement into your spine.

TAKE NOTE

- Rate the difficulty 1–10.
- Which hand / arm position feels most comfortable for you?
- Can you straighten your arms?
- Where do you feel a stretch: Abs? Back?
- Any issues? If so, where?

- Pay attention to how your body feels when you're in this position and note exactly where it feels tight or 'not quite right' – the more detail the merrier.

Once you've wiggled your way to warmth, we're going to take this up a notch from a passive stretch to an active hold.

CHALLENGE TWO: SAUCY COBRA

Start by setting up for your cobra again, only this time unpoint your ballerina toes and press them into the floor, as you would for a push up. As you lift your chest off the ground, bring your hips with you so only your hands and toes are in contact with the floor. Tense your glutes, pull back your shoulders, and inhale that sweet, sweet oxygen. Aim to hold this position for five big, deep breaths (roughly 30 seconds) without crumbling to the floor. Lifting your hips off the ground turns this gentle passive stretch into a strengthening exercise at the same time. And if there's one thing we love, it's a move that stretches and strengthens at the same time.

If this is a little too much for the ol' spine to begin with, just stick to what feels manageable for you for now, and whenever you slide into your cobra, see if you can lift that little bit further or hold that little bit longer over time.

Why the Cobra?

Throughout these challenges you've moved your spine in every possible way, from the Jefferson curl to touching your toes (flexion), side plank lifts (lateral flexion) and holds (resisting movement), to the world's greatest stretch (rotation). The cobra completes this quartet with a little extension. If you want to keep the 33 joints that make up your spine nice and healthy (which you certainly do), I believe it's a good idea to expose it to the widest possible range of movements, to keep your saucy spine flowing and prepare you for the random movements that come with moving your way through life. The cobra is one of the simplest ways of working some back extension into your life without any equipment.

I'm sure I don't need to remind you, but don't forget to have a wiggle while you're getting your snake on. Roll your shoulders forwards and back, twist your head to look over towards your toes, and explore where feels a little stiff or a little tender. This is your opportunity to play. And if you want to take it up another mobility notch, then it's time to get your flow on.

Flow Baby Flow

While this isn't just specific to the cobra, this move provides a lovely segue into movement flows. Though I've introduced the exercises in these challenges as stand-alone, they don't have to sit on their own all the time; some of them can be thrown together in a sort of mobility combo by flowing from one to the other.

BONUS CHALLENGE: COBRA DOG FLOW

If you're unsure of what I mean by a movement flow, start in your cobra position. Hold for a breath, then push your hips back to transition into a downward dog. Oi oi, you just did a little flow – spicy, huh?

The flow doesn't have to stop there. If you want to take the spice level from jalapeño up to habanero, come down from the dog and bust a push up, before getting your leg up and wiggling into the world's greatest stretch. Now you're really flowing and the possibilities are endless.

You don't always have to turn a move into a flow to get the best out of it, but every now and again, playing around and combining a few exercises is a great way of getting more movement variety into a short space of time, especially if you haven't had the chance to get much movement into your day and you're feeling a little stiff. Playing with movement pairings is a delightful way of sprinkling some mobility novelty into your life and spicing things up every now and then.

Whenever, Wherever

I'm all for encouraging you to bust these moves out whenever and wherever. But I appreciate lying down on the floor in the middle of the day isn't always the easiest, or the most 'socially acceptable'. Although I deep down hope you wouldn't let that stop you. So, if you're keen to squeeze this spinal manoeuvre into your day, there's few better places than the comfort of your own bed when you wake in the morning and just before you got to sleep. I don't think there's much better ways to start a day than with a sprinkle of purposeful movement, and you might just find that once you've bust out this one move, that more start to follow. Before you know it, you'll have banked some cheeky movement minutes before your day's even started.

You Scratch Your Back and I'll Scratch Mine: Apley Scratch Test

Ideal for: Shoulders (Internal Rotation, Extension, External Rotation, Flexion)

Sick of leaving that one spot on your back perpetually unwashed? Tired of missing that tiny area of un-sun-creamed skin on your back because you just can't reach and don't fancy asking a stranger to rub your back? Fed up with not being able to scratch that elusive itch in between your shoulder blades? Today, we say 'no more', as we *finally* learn how to touch our hands behind our backs (or at least get closer).

Welcome to the 'Hands Behind Your Back' challenge, also known as the Apley Scratch Test, where, you've guessed it, we'll test your ability to touch your hands behind your back! Here, you will learn a simple trick that will help improve the function of your shoulders, specifically their ability to rotate externally and internally, but before I show you how, let's see how close you are to finger-locking goodness already.

To save you the trouble of trying to look behind you while you attempt to touch fingertips, this is another gentle reminder to WHIP OUT YOUR CAMERA and record yourself.

CHALLENGE ONE:
TOUCH YOUR HANDS BEHIND YOUR BACK

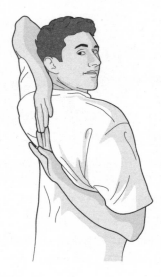

Reaching one hand above your head and the other behind your back, I want you to see how close you can get your fingers to each other.

Once you've attempted this on one side, try the other.

TAKE NOTE

- Rate the difficulty 1–10.
- Can you do this on both sides? Just one side? Neither?
- Is one side easier than the other? If so, which?
- Any issues? If so, where?
- Pay attention to how your body feels when you're in this position and note exactly where it feels tight or 'not quite right' – the more detail the merrier.

If you found yourself wondering 'when does the challenge begin?' as you gracefully interlocked your fingers on both sides with ease, then it looks like you're not lacking in shoulder flexibility, especially in the external and internal rotation department. For someone of your current shoulder bendiness, you may not need to focus too much on improving these areas of flexibility, unless you have outlandish mobility hopes and dreams. Just keep greasing those shoulder grooves and checking in on these abilities regularly.

However, if you found yourself struggling on one or both sides, I've got a simple method to help you improve, and a spicy way of sliding this into your life – *win win*. But first, let's look at what this move tells us about your shoulders.

External and Internal Rotation

To get your hands meeting behind your back requires a few movement abilities to be up to scratch. The overhead arm requires flexion to bring the arm up, and external rotation to twist it behind your head; while the behind your back arm needs to extend behind you and internally rotate to tickle the shoulder blades. To better understand what external and internal rotation is, I want you to imagine you and I are having an arm wrestle. If you win, you end up in internal rotation, if you lose you finish externally rotated. When touching your hands behind your back, you need a certain amount of both.

Let me guess, you found it harder to internally rotate your right hand behind your back than you did your left hand, didn't you? If you're wondering how I knew that, I need to come clean. This isn't some Derren Brown mind trick. The truth is, I only had two hands to choose from, so I'm bound to choose the winner at least half of the time, right? Based on my experience, it seems the odds are slightly skewed from a 50–50 split with a higher percentage of us finding it harder to get our right hand behind your back because of the natural, asymmetrical shape of our skeleton.

On the surface, it looks like we're pretty symmetrical, but under the hood we're not quite so split down the middle, with our left-leaning heart, right-leaning diaphragm, and one boob or bollock that often hangs lower than the other. Our skeleton is no different (at least for most of us). A decent proportion of us will find our right shoulder sits slightly lower and further forwards than our left, making it harder to get the right hand behind our back. If this is you, it will mean your right shoulder blade is more likely to 'wing' than its opposing partner on the left-hand side. A winged shoulder blade is one that doesn't quite sit flush on your ribcage, and for years I was led to believe that this was a dysfunction and likely to lead to shoulder problems. If you too have a winged or wonky scapular, I come bearing good news, as research suggests that this asymmetry in resting positions and movement is normal.[1] So, if your shoulders feel fine, don't worry if they're not 100 per cent symmetrical! While this isn't a strict rule of anatomy, and plenty of variation exists among us, it may give you some insight as to why some of you find it more difficult to touch your hands behind your back on one side than the other. Simply put: we're not symmetrical, and that's okay.

For some of us, no matter how good our external and internal rotation, our hands will never meet like this due to the structure of the bones in your shoulders. If you're a larger human or have shorter arms, you too may find it difficult. However, before you rule yourself out of ever back-handedly tickling those fingers together, know that you can still benefit from improving this ability, even without the hand-to-hand connection. So don't throw in the towel just yet – because you're going to need it.

The Tea Towel Trick

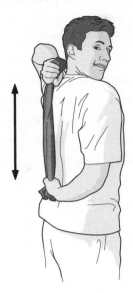

To improve shoulder flexibility in this position and gradually work your fingers closer together, you're going to need a tea towel (or any kind of towel). This towel works by bridging the gap between your hands and helping you pull your shoulders deeper into the stretch. For the sake of this book, we're going to call this the 'hands behind your back floss'.

Starting with the towel in the hand that goes above your head, fling it over your shoulder and grab hold of it with the hand reaching up behind your back. You should feel a light stretch, but it shouldn't be so intense that it feels like your bone is going to fly out of its socket. If you're struggling, grab a longer towel (or even a T-shirt or rope). Once your chosen prop is firmly in both hands, you're going to gently floss up and down, with your top hand pulling your bottom hand higher up your back, going to the point at which you feel the stretch. At this point, I want you to stop, take a big, deep breath, nice and slowly, then pull and do the exact same thing in the opposite direction, with the bottom hand pulling the top hand downwards. The more time you spend in this position, the more your body will get used to it and the easier it will become.

Using your breath is going to be really useful here, helping you to get deeper into the stretch by expanding your ribs, but also by helping you relax further into the stretch.

By now, hopefully you've started to realise that this book is all about finding ways to squeeze these moves into your life. Next time you're in the kitchen cooking or cleaning up, take a minute or two to floss your hands behind your back. If this becomes a regular feature in your day, your hands will be best behind-the-back buds in no time. And the move doesn't have to stay in the kitchen – you can give it a go when you get in and out of the shower, or while you're doing the laundry . . . Get creative! Just make sure you don't rush or force the stretch. I believe the best strategy here is regularity rather than intensity. And before you know it, you might even be able to scratch that elusive itch.

W to Y: Prone Press

Ideal for: Upper Back, Neck, Shoulders

Feel a 'knot' in between or around your shoulder blades? Or a constant tight feeling in your upper back? Well, this move might just be the answer. I need you to kiss the carpet to get into position for the Prone Press, and lie face down on the floor. We're about to get your back and shoulders working together with this simple-looking yet delightfully challenging move known as the prone press, or W to Y raise.

Expect to feel all of the muscles in your back working overtime with this juicy number. You won't *need* any equipment, but if you do have some small weights or a resistance band, I'll show you how to milk a little more out of the move.

You're probably bored of me saying it by now, but in case you haven't already, WHIP OUT YOUR CAMERA and get recording.

CHALLENGE ONE: PRONE PRESS

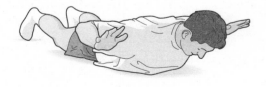

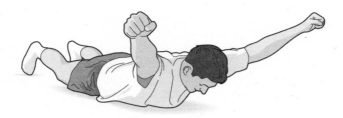

Start lying face down on the floor (known as a 'prone' position). If you don't have a floor with enough space, you can lie face down on your bed. Once prone, stretch your arms above your head, as if you're doing the 'Y' in YMCA, with palms facing the floor (or bed). From here, lift everything from your chest up off the floor (shoulders, head, arms, etc.) while keeping your belly in contact with the floor. Squeeze your glutes, then pull your elbows towards your hips, until your upper arm is caressing your ribcage (or at least close), making a sort of W shape with your arms if you were looking from a bird's eye view. Hold this W for a big breath, and then slowly reach your arms back into your Y shape, with as much control as possible (the slower the better). Once back in your Y, lower your chest, head and arms to the floor. Boom, the prone press.

You can also start in the W shape and raise to the Y; it's just a lot easier to describe it the other way around! Give both a go.

TAKE NOTE

- Rate the difficulty 1–10.
- Were you able to complete the movement in one smooth transition?
- Which muscles do you feel working the most? Upper back? Lower back? Shoulders? Neck?

- Any issues? If so, where?
- Pay attention to how your body feels when you're in this position and note exactly where it feels tight or 'not quite right' – the more detail the merrier.

When it comes to training with little to no equipment, it can be hard to get the back muscles working, but this move tickles some of those difficult to reach places. A great aim here is to be able to complete 10–20 repetitions, slow and controlled, from W to Y (or Y to W), but don't worry too much about the numbers. To get the most bang for your buck, I want you moving super slow, like never before. This move is all about building control between the two points (W to Y), not rushing through the movement. One rep that takes 10 seconds is better than 10 reps that last one second. The key is to spend as much 'time under tension', which simply refers to how long our muscles spend working throughout the exercise, and will really help challenge your ability to control the muscles across your back and shoulders.

TUBA (Tight Upper Back Alert)

For a large part of my mid-twenties, I had this seemingly unshakable stiffness across my upper back that felt like a 'knot' between my shoulder blades. I won't lie, I have no idea what that knot sensation actually is, but after years of searching for a remedy, I stumbled across this gem and it has become my go-to whenever that tight feeling creeps its way back into my life – especially after long periods curled up at a computer (in other words, the entire time I've been writing this book). Obviously, this move isn't a one-size-fits-all, and I can't guarantee that it will work for you as it did for me. But if you are struggling with a constant stiff feeling across your upper back, you have nothing to lose. Give this move a go and let me know if it helps.

Once you've done as many W to Y raises as you can, relax but stay in this prone position, with your arms in the W shape resting on the floor, and take 5–10 (or however many you want) slow, gentle, deep breaths. With each breath you should feel your ribcage expand and a nice stretch in the muscles across your upper back. Just try and relax with each breath; remember, we don't want to fight tension with more tension.

This approach of strengthening and then actively relaxing any tight areas or muscles has worked wonders for me, and I'm hoping it will for you too.

Adaptations

Lying on your front can be uncomfortable for some people. If this is you, you can achieve a similar result by standing up and leaning forward by hinging your hips backwards (see page 79 for your hinge reminder). The reason lying down works so well is that it takes our lower body out of the equation and allows us to challenge the shoulders and back more directly. When you hinge and lean forwards, your lower back will work to keep you there, and that area may tire before your shoulders and back. However, if needed, it will still work. Alternatively, if your lower back doesn't agree with that, you can try kneeling down and sitting back on your heels, if your lower body mobility allows. This is a viable option to getting some upper back and shoulder movement.

If you have access to a gym-style bench, you can set the bench to an incline that suits you and repeat the exact same thing, with the general rule of thumb that the more horizontal you are, the harder the move, and the more upright the easier. You can even benefit from doing this movement standing up, if hinging over or lying down just isn't an option. All you need to do is stand with your back against a wall and transition between the W and Y position while trying to keep as much of your upper body in contact with the wall as possible. Imagine you're performing a sort of anticlimactic wall snow angel.

If these all feel a tad too easy for you and you have some small weights lying around, slap them in your hands and give it a go – you won't need much weight for a spicy stimulus here. Or if you have a resistance band, you can hold that in your hands as you move between the W and Y positions. Having some tension on the band adds a unique stimulus that you don't get with just your arms or light weights, as it engages the muscles around your shoulders a little differently. So, if you have one lying around the house, give it a go!

If you find working both arms at the same time a tad too demanding, you can ease up a little by trying one arm at a time, either face down or while lying on your side, propped up by your other elbow. This will help if you have a big discrepancy in mobility between arms. Play around and find what suits you.

Can't Move from W to Y?

If waving your arms above your head like you just don't care feels far from possible at the moment, maybe your arms just don't want to move that way? So, instead of transitioning between both positions, I want you to break it down into just Ws and just Ys.

Spend time practising lifting your arms from the floor into both positions to help build strength in those back muscles of yours. This will help you build up to the transitions over time.

When you can manage up to 20 controlled lifts in both the W and Y position, I guarantee you'll find it a lot easier to reintroduce the transition between the two.

If you find getting into the Y shape impossible no matter what you do, first try working on your shoulder dislocates (page 147) and downward dogs (page 155). These will hopefully improve your ability to get your arms above your head before we start strengthening them a little more.

It's a Trap, a Lower Trap!

One of the major benefits of this exercise is its ability to target a muscle that sits in the middle of your back, known on the street as the lower traps. The trapezius is a rather large muscle that starts at the base of your skull and spans your entire upper back, across your shoulders and down to the middle of your spine in the shape of a kite (or a diamond, or trapezoid shape, which I had no idea was a thing until I googled it). Although one big muscle, it's often categorised into three sections, upper, middle and lower, based on the direction of the muscle fibres and the role they play. While I'm not going to test you on it, what you do need to know is that this muscle plays a huge role in supporting you as a two-legged human with a head, specifically by helping to stabilise your scapula, so it's a good idea to get it moving and strengthen it from time to time, and this move does just that.

Not only does this move challenge those lower traps of yours, but it also challenges loads of other juicy muscles on your back, such as the rhomboids, rear delts, rotator cuff muscles around your shoulders, and the muscles all the way up your neck. And as the final cherry on the cake, it's a wicked opportunity to defrost from your prawn posture after a long day curled up at your desk.

Push It Real Good: The Push Up

Ideal for: Chest, Shoulders, Arms, Wrists, Core

It's time to push it real good, with this absolute classic. There aren't many simpler or more effective ways of building upper body strength than a good ol' push up. While the idea of lowering and pushing your bodyweight up from the floor may seem intimidating at first, the aim here is to show you that it doesn't have to be – *and* that there are plenty of rewards to be reaped even without the ability to do a full push up.

In this challenge we'll explore your current pushing capabilities and how to find a level that suits you, while building towards your first full bodyweight push up. If you've always secretly wanted to be able to do a push up, then I'm going to do everything I can to help you realise your ambition. But first, let's see what you've got.

You know what I'm going to say, don't you? WHIP OUT YOUR CAMERA!

CHALLENGE ONE: A PUSH UP

Most of you will be familiar with this movement, or at least the idea of it. So, all I want you to do is drop down to the floor and give your best attempt at a bodyweight push up. The bonus of this exercise is that it requires nothing but a floor, a body and gravity.

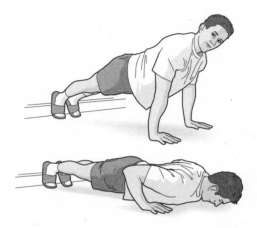

Before I give you any pointers, set yourself up in a position that feels natural for you to do a push up. Supported by the palms of your hands and tips of your toes, with your arms straight and hips and knees off the ground, get into the shape of the illustration above, if you can. From here, attempt to lower yourself to the ground with as much control as possible, as low as you can without quite touching the floor, then push yourself back up to the top again.

TAKE NOTE

- Rate the difficulty 1–10.
- Are you able to do a full push up?
- How low can you go? All the way down? Halfway? Just an inch?
- What about the way up?
- Which muscles do you feel working the most?
- Any issues? If so, where?
- Pay attention to how your body feels when you're in this position and note exactly where it feels tight or 'not quite right' – the more detail the merrier.

If you were able to thrust your chest from the floor with ease, then give yourself a round of applause, because a push up is an incredible feat of strength that I wholeheartedly believe we should all aim to master if we want to build a mobile body.

If you found your forehead aggressively kissing the carpet, then please don't give up hope. You may not be able to do a push up just yet, but the key word in that sentence is *yet.* I assure you, this is a skill worth pursuing.

What's So Good About a Push Up?

Apart from being able to show off your shiny new skill and fend someone off with a strong shove, there are loads of benefits to being able to lower your body to the floor in a controlled manner and push it back up again. Let's start with the most obvious.

Fall Protection

Falls again, really? Some things can be mentioned once and never again, but with as many as 37.3 million falls being severe enough to require medical attention globally each year, this ain't one of them.[1] I don't want to inject any unnecessary fear into your life, but the stats don't lie. Being the second leading cause of unintentional death worldwide (I'm sure you're immediately wondering what's number one – it's road traffic injuries), anything we can do to reduce the risk of falls or reduce the severity of injury from falls is a worthwhile pursuit, and working to improve our push up ability will do just that. After all, this push up business has as much to do with lowering ourselves down with control as it does with actually pushing ourselves up, so working on our strength and mobility in this area is a surefire way to help protect you if you do ever fall head over heels (and not in the good way).

Full Body Strength and Stability

The push up requires strength in your upper body in order to lower yourself down with control and push yourself back up again, without just flopping onto the floor. To finesse this strength-building beauty, it requires your hands, wrists, arms, shoulders and chest to work together to resist gravity's pull while generating enough force to propel you from the floor. This harmonious push from the upper body relies especially on the stability of the shoulders. This stability is assisted by your rotator cuff muscles and your shoulder blades, which is why it's important to keep them strong, so they are able to move freely across your ribcage as you move up and down.

Beyond the more obvious upper body involvement, a solid push up needs the *whole* body to work together as one big chain, engaging the muscles in the back, core, glutes, and all the way down to the legs, to stop you collapsing onto the deck. This means we get a huge bang for our buck from such a *simple movement.* Getting stronger, while at the same time learning how to move our whole body in harmony as one unit – lovely. In the beginning, this whole-body tension will probably feel quite intense, but as you get stronger and more coordinated, your body won't have to work as hard, and you'll feel how much easier it is to glide up and down.

You might be thinking: 'Simple?! Adam, it's impossible!' And sure, it may feel that way at the moment. If you've never practised, this move can be one hell of a challenge – but that's a good thing, because it's meant to be! If you're struggling to push yourself up, you've got so much to gain. This could be the key you've been looking for.

The Incline Push Up

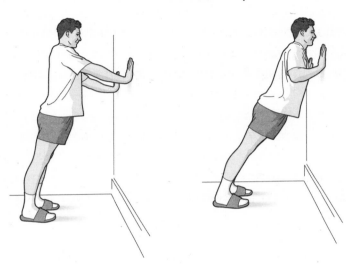

The good news is that you don't have to start from the ground in order to soak up all the goodness of this position, as it's easy to adapt. Say hello to the incline push up. If starting from the floor is simply too difficult, you can introduce an 'incline' by making sure your shoulders are higher than your feet, while keeping your feet on the ground. This change in orientation makes the movement much easier – the more upright you are, the less intense the push up will be. You can get creative and use whatever suits you best: by placing your hands on a wall, a kitchen countertop or table, or my personal favourite, the stairs. Over time, as you get stronger, more confident and comfortable with the movement, you can progress onto lower structures (using a lower step, for example) until you're feeling strong enough to take to the floor again, hopefully less head-on this time.

As with all of these exercises, there's no magic number, but here's a simple blueprint to follow to work your way up (or down) to a push up from the floor.

Find a surface on which you can perform between 5 and 15 good-quality push ups. By quality, I simply mean controlled, not bouncing like a yo-yo. The slower the movement downwards, the more time under tension and the harder your muscles have to work. There's nothing wrong with doing more than 15 – in fact, if you can, brilliant! Between 5 and 15 is simply a guide, and a nice middle ground amount that's not so challenging that you lose control of the movement and burst a vein in your forehead, but not so little that it doesn't make a difference. Once you've nailed 15, you should be confident that you have enough strength to reduce the incline. The aim is to repeat this process again and again on progressively lower surfaces until you're a fully-fledged member of the push up club.

I can't tell you exactly how long this will take, as everyone's different, but if you follow this simple approach and practise regularly – even as little as 2–3 times a week – you can build enough mobility and strength to smash out your first ever push up. I've seen it happen with my own clients; the transformation can be incredible! Before you know it, you'll forget you ever struggled. Just don't feel the need to rush to move on to lower surfaces. As long as you're practising regularly and improving over time, you're doing a phenomenal job.

Mobility Snack:
Find Your Personal Push Up Stations

We've all got little areas in our house that are perfect for mini bursts of exercise. And once we label them clearly in our mind – or literally, with a Post-It note or giant neon sign – integrating movement into our day becomes a lot easier. Right this minute (unless you're reading this on a train or something!) is your chance to find your push up station. For me, it's my kitchen countertop and my stairs. Whenever I'm waiting for something to cook, the kettle to boil, or walking up the stairs, I get this annoying voice like a devil (or angel) on my shoulder, nagging, 'Go on, Adam, do some push ups.' And before I know it, I've done 30 and got my heart pumping while giving my chest a nice little stretch. Find a couple of places in your house, at work, *anywhere*, that you can designate as your personal push up station and get pushing!

Our ability to drop and bust out push ups on command (or at will) is linked with a reduced risk of heart disease, which I think we can all agree is a positive. Research suggests that those who can comfortably perform push ups are significantly less likely to develop heart disease compared to those who can do very few, or none at all.[2] Once you've built up to a few sets of 15+ push ups and felt your heart working overtime, you'll see why! Not only is this exercise an incredible strength and stability builder across the shoulders and the rest of the body, when we start to build up to larger repetitions, we're able to challenge the heart's stamina and ability to supply blood to the muscles to keep them working. And if there's one thing a mobile body needs, it's a strong heart. So, what you waiting for? You don't need to drop and give me 20 just yet. Instead, why not lean and give me 10? The important thing is that you're getting your muscles moving, heart pumping, joints lubing and aiming to get stronger over time.

How Do I Do a Push Up?

If you search how to do a push up online, you'll be bombarded with videos and explanations of the 'right' and 'wrong' ways of doing it. I'm not convinced it's that simple. While there will be tips and tricks that will help to make the movement easier for you, our bodies are unique and move in lots of weird and wonderful ways. I operate under the belief that it's best to start with what feels natural to you, rather than obsessing over minute details of technique that probably don't matter as much as some people suggest.

What's for sure is that the position of your hands will distribute the forces in different places. Arms further out to the side, in line with your shoulders (in an almost T-shape) will stretch your shoulders and chest more, whereas arms closer to your torso will require more effort from your triceps (back of your arms). Some may find it easier to progress with their hands wide, others will find it less gnarly with their arms closer together. There are no set movement rules around here! So, take this as your licence to play, be your own scientist and find what feels best for you.

My Wrists Hurt!

If you've played around with the placement of your hands but it's still hurting your wrists, it may be worth working on your wrist mobility. Here's a quick routine you can try to see if it helps.

1. Start by clasping your hands together – hold your hands in prayer position, then interlock your fingers and twirl your hands in different directions. Do this for 30 seconds to get everything nice and warmed up.
2. Get on all fours with your hands and knees on the floor. Rock your weight forwards gently until you feel a stretch in your wrists/forearms. Hold for 5 seconds then rock back. Repeat this 6–10 times, then rest for 30 seconds.

3. Get back on all fours with hands on the floor. While pressing your fingers into the ground, lift the heels of your hands off the floor and gently lower back down. You should feel this all down your forearm. Do this 6–10 times.

4. Retest your push up and see if it feels any better. It may help to repeat the steps above a couple of times and, if you feel an immediate benefit, follow them regularly before you bust out your push ups.

If your wrists still hurt, it's worth investigating further with a medical professional. But in the meantime, you can still practise your push ups by adapting your wrist position. Try placing a towel under the heels of your hands to make the movement less intense on your wrist. Alternatively, you can try doing push ups on your fists or while holding on to handles of dumbbells, or something similar. This should take the immediate strain off of your wrist while you work on improving your wrist mobility.

Shoulder Stability and Scapula Control

Your shoulder is one hell of a contraption. This wild joint has a lot going on under the hood that allows it to travel around all over the shop, but one thing it needs to function healthily is a good control of the shoulder blade (scapula). This little 'blade' of bone sits on the back of our ribcage and glides up, down and side to side as we move our shoulder. But without sufficient coordination and control of this bone, we can easily lose out on shoulder mobility. The push up gives us a sensational opportunity to shine a spotlight on our shoulders' number one supporter and make sure it's working well. We can also complement the move with a little addition to really test our blades.

When you lower yourself down in a push up, your shoulder blades retract, moving closer to your spine. As you push yourself up, they protract, moving outwards, around your ribcage and towards your shoulders. This happens as a 'natural' response to the movement to maintain stability in your shoulders. Next time you push yourself up, when you get to the top position, I want you to round your upper back, as if you're trying to get as much distance between your chest and the floor without moving your hands. This will allow your shoulder blades to protract as far as they can. Try not to 'shrug' and lift your shoulders up towards your ears. Instead, think about spreading your shoulder blades as far apart as possible when you can't go any further, then pause and lower yourself down again. This extra scapula spice is going to go a long way in helping to maintain healthy, happy shoulders.

What's Next?

If you've mastered the push up and it feels all too easy for you now, the next step is raising your hands on a platform, like two workout benches, two dumbbells or two stools, to allow your chest to drop below your hands in the bottom of the push up; this is known as a 'deficit' push up. You'll feel an incredible stretch in your chest and shoulders, due to the extra challenge to the position of your shoulder joints, helping build strength and improving your end-range flexibility at the same time.

CHANGE PLACES. You know exactly why by now!

On All Fours: Tabletop

*Ideal for: Shoulders, Wrists,
Pecs, Biceps, Glutes, Abdominals*

I adore this exercise. It ticks so many mobility boxes and doubles up as both a strength and stretch movement. If I can get two birds for my stone, I'm having 'em. When you first get into this position, you'll experience a deep stretch across the front of your shoulders, chest and into your biceps. It's technically an incredible shoulder strength and stability sculpting exercise, but you'll also challenge your core and your gluteus maximus – *all in one go*. Finally, I'm a fan because you'll look like a crab while doing it and I just personally think that's funny.

In case you're struggling to imagine what this movement looks like, take a glance at the illustrations overleaf, or even better, follow my instructions before you try to give it a whirl yourself. Just don't forget to WHIP OUT YOUR CAMERA, because you're definitely going to want to see this one – not just to appreciate your crab impression, but to see your progress over time too.

CHALLENGE: THE TABLETOP

Pop yourself down on the floor, sitting on your butt, with your knees bent at roughly 90 degrees (no need to whip out the protractor, roughly is fine). Your hands should be on the floor behind

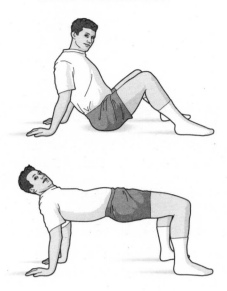

you, fingers facing away from your body, towards the wall behind you. This is your set up position.

Once here, lift your hips off the floor, as high as you can, as if you're trying to make a tabletop with your body (we love it when the name of the exercise makes sense). Hold this position for as many controlled breaths as you can, then lower yourself down.

TAKE NOTE

- Rate the difficulty 1–10.
- Are you able to get all the way up, with your body parallel with the floor?
- How many breaths can you take before lowering down?
- Where do you feel the movement the most?
- Any issues? If so, where?

- Pay attention to how your body feels when you're in this position and note exactly where it feels tight or 'not quite right' – the more detail the merrier.

Can't Get it Up All the Way?

This is such a common problem, and one nobody should be ashamed of. As always, it just means there's an opportunity for growth and that we've found something to work on and improve. Just as we have done with any kind of struggle in these movement challenges, start by dialling things back. I think it really helps to know that you will still be able to progress, just by pushing your hips as high as you can. Wherever that is, take a breath, then lower down and repeat this as many times as you can until it feels around an 8/10 intensity. At this point, stop and take a rest. If you still have some more juice, you can repeat the process for 1–3 more rounds, depending on how you feel or how much time you have. Each time you practise, you'll find it a little easier to push a smidge higher as you get stronger and more flexible. You never know – this could soon be your favourite mobility moment, and you might even find yourself busting this crabby move out as your newest party trick. To speed along the process, it may help to open up the front side of your body by spending a little more time practising the couch stretch (page 114), hip flexor lunge (page 119) and cobra (page 162).

What's So Special about the Tabletop?

Apart from how funny it looks, this move is the only one in this entire series that focuses on extending our shoulders behind us. In doing so, it helps us feel that intense stretch across our chest, shoulders and arms, while also building strength at the same time. For most of us living curled up at our desks or over our phones or books 24/7 like prawns, opening up the front of our body more regularly is going to feel really bloody good. I'm sure I don't need to tell you how amazing it feels to get a stretch across the front of the shoulders after being sat down for a long time. So if you haven't tried this one already, this is the time to get your butt on the floor and bust out your best tabletop impression.

Building on the Tabletop

Once you feel confident that you could pass as a legitimate coffee table, I want you to add some play into the movement and get wiggling around a little. Explore how it feels when you lift one leg off the ground, and then the other. What happens if you lift one hand off the ground? Or try to walk about like a crab in this position? There are no set rules when it comes to how we move, so just use this tabletop exercise as a template and build on it. There's so much benefit to just playing with these positions and breaking free from the basic A to B I've outlined at the top of this challenge.

Feels So Good But Hurts So Bad

If the stretch feels sensational but the move is a little too intense on your wrists, or maybe your shoulders just don't bend that way no matter how hard you try, here's a chair-based suggestion to get your stretch on but without having to get your crab on. As much as I love this move, I can appreciate it isn't the most practical if you're in the middle of a busy office, even if it would be funny to watch. While sat on your chair, reach your arms behind you and prop them on top of the backrest of the chair. If the chair's a little too big, start standing. Once your arms are firmly propped, lift your chest up, tall and proud, until you feel a stretch across your front and down your arms. When you've held the position for 30 seconds, or for a few big, deep breaths, relax and repeat as many times as you like. I won't lie, I have no idea what this is called, but we'll call it the chair chest stretch. That works, right?

If your wrists were the culprit for the lack of tabletopping, it might also be worth practising some lighter weight-bearing moves such as incline push ups (page 183) and downward dogs (page 153) before giving the tabletop another bash and spend some time practising the mini wrist mobility routine on page 186.

Let's Hang: Dead Hang

*Ideal for: Hands (Grip), Wrists, Forearms,
Shoulders, Upper Back, Lats*

This book wouldn't be complete without an ode to our fuzzy ancestor, the chimpanzee. It's weird to think we descended from the trees all those years ago and spent such a large proportion of our evolutionary history monkeying around and swinging about. I'm a fan of our modern world, so there's no need to regress back through time, become one with nature and literally climb a tree for this challenge (although I would love it if you did). However, you *will* need to find some kind of bar to dangle from for this champion challenge! Whether that means scoping out a public pull up bar, buying one for your home that you can fit over a door frame, popping to the gym, or simply getting creative with what you have around you, it will absolutely be worth the effort.

In this challenge I'm going to teach you why hanging is one of the most incredible things you can do for your mobility, and why grip strength is a strong predictor of how long you'll live.

As always, we'll adapt the exercise for your needs and guide you on how to build up strength over time, but for now it's time to see what you've got in the locker already!

You're going to make me remind you again, aren't you? Okay, fine. WHIP OUT YOUR CAMERA, it's recording time.

CHALLENGE ONE: THE DEAD HANG

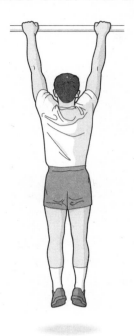

The 'dead hang' might sound a tad dramatic, but it's not as life or death as it sounds (or is it . . . ?). Find a bar, grab hold and hang for as long as you can without your feet touching the floor.

If you're wondering how to hold on to the bar, there are a few grip options.

- Overhand or pronated (palms away from you)
- Underhand or supinated (palms towards you)
- Neutral (palms facing each other – if your pull up bar allows it!)
- Commando (one hand over, one hand under)

While these different grips will challenge your muscles in slightly different ways by changing the position of your hands, it doesn't really matter which you use, so try not to over-complicate it, just play around and find what's comfortable for you.

TAKE NOTE

- Rate the difficulty 1–10.
- How long can you hang for?
- Where do you feel the stretch the most?
- Which grip feels best?
- Any issues? If so, where?
- Pay attention to how your body feels when you're in this position and note exactly where it feels tight or 'not quite right' – the more detail the merrier.

There's no definitive time you need to hang for. The important thing is that you improve over time. I won't be totally vague and leave you without a warm fuzzy feeling and a dopamine-inducing pat on the back for your dangling-based achievements, however, so here are some time-based accolades to strive for:

10 SECONDS

Working up to your first 10 seconds can often be the hardest, especially if you're a complete beginner, so if you passed the 10-second mark – well done! This is your foundation and, once you get here, building on it becomes easier and easier.

30 SECONDS

Once you cross the 30-second mark you're literally halfway to a minute and well on your way to dangling proficiency, demonstrating solid strength. Keep going – 1 minute is on the horizon.

60 SECONDS

Does gravity even exist anymore?! Well . . . yes, but you're doing a good job at fighting against it! This is a smashing milestone in the hanging Olympics, and you should be incredibly proud. Nicolas Cage has been in touch, and he wants to recruit you for his upcoming film *Still Here After 60 Seconds*. (If you don't get the reference, google it – though you're not missing much.)

2 MINUTES

Hot diggity damn! You're at one with the bar. Chances are there'll rarely be a time you'll need to dangle from anything for longer than 2 minutes, unless you care to dip your toe into the world of rock climbing and find yourself hanging off a cliff edge. However, this shows an incredible level of grip strength and stamina.

Strong Hands Save Lives

'Could a strong set of mitts really save my life?' you may ask. And the answer would be *yes*. But the reasons why might surprise you. Believe it or not, low grip strength has been consistently linked with increased risk of kicking the bucket a little prematurely, and there are loads of reasons why, some more obvious than others.

Fall Protection

Let's face it, the chances of you dangling off the edge of a cliff and fighting for survival are low, but when it comes to taking a tumble, it's a lot more common than you might think. Our ability to balance will always be our best line of defence when it comes to falling, as prevention is better than reaction, but a strong grip is a sensational backup. No matter how good your balance, we all fall from time to time.

If you've ever taken a tumble and found yourself flailing instinctively to grab on to anything in your immediate vicinity, you'll appreciate the importance of a sturdy grip when it comes to saving your bacon. Swift reactions and strong digits can make the world of difference, by reducing the impact of falls and helping to turn a nasty trip into a light bump on the head rather than a trip to the hospital. This becomes especially useful as we get older, when muscle wastage (known as sarcopenia) becomes a reality. It makes sense that a strong grip can protect against falls, right? But a strong grip can also reveal a lot more about our overall health.

The Hidden Benefits of a Strong Grip

A strong grip has consistently been shown to reduce your risk of dying from *all causes*.[1] While I'd love to imagine this means that if I hang and carry enough heavy shopping bags, my hands will develop powers similar to that of Harry Potter waving his wand.

Sadly it doesn't. This miraculous link is less to do with the direct benefits of strong hands, and more about what it indicates about your lifestyle.

Simply put, a strong grip is a likely indicator of an active life, and we all know the benefits of being an active little bean. There are countless studies exploring the link between grip strength and longevity, suggesting the stronger your grip (within reason), the more likely your overall strength, upper limb function, bone density, nutritional status, cognitive abilities, heart health and overall quality of life are to be in decent working order.[2] It's also been noted that elderly people with significantly lower grip strength are more likely to struggle with basic mobility, such as standing up, walking, and generally getting up and about.[3] Although our hands might not be magic, it's fair to say these fingers are pretty bloody useful, especially if we keep them nice and strong, and it's a good idea to do so if you want to live a long, healthy life.

Why Hang?

There are plenty of incredible ways to train your grip. Simply picking up and holding some heavy things will do a grand job of working the fingers and all the forearm muscles involved in your grip, but when it comes to all-round benefit, hanging will always be my go-to, because of the three things which are hard to get elsewhere when looking beyond just grip strength.

Stretch, Strength and Stability

By now you've hopefully been converted to my fictional mobility church, and primed as a keen mobility missionary eager to preach the benefits of a strong, stable and bendy body. Thus, when faced with an opportunity to tick all three boxes in one move, we need to grab it by the horns and hold on to it for dear life. Which, ironically, will be a lot easier with a stronger grip.

Not only does this incredibly simple activity yield marvellous results for your grip strength and general wellbeing, dangling also gives us a unique opportunity to stretch and strengthen the shoulders at the same time.

For everyone currently sat at their laptop like my favourite pink crustacean, this is another one for you. While I've already told you that sitting in a rounded shape isn't necessarily a terrible thing, spending long periods in this prawn-like posture (also known as kyphosis or kyphotic) means that this thoracic part of the spine doesn't move very much, and our arms rarely go above our heads. By now we know that motion is lotion. So, finding ways to extend the thorax (ribcage), lift our arms above our head and push our chest out to the world is going to be useful for opening up all the muscles that help us breathe, move our shoulders and exist as a functioning human. Sprinkle that with a strength activity and we're on to a winner, hence why I believe the hang rules supreme.

You'll also likely notice a deep stretch sensation underneath your armpits and all the way down the side of your back. That big muscle you're feeling is known as the latissimus dorsi (the lats). This rather large muscle inserts at your armpits and covers almost the entire back, and is responsible for extending your arms as you bring them from overhead, down by your side and behind your back. This muscle can also be responsible for restricting your arms from going above your head if they're a little stiff.

Adam, Man, I Can't Hang!

Oh but you can, my dear friend, and you shall! We just need to adapt the movement, and here's how.

If you're unable to dangle from your bar without losing your grip almost instantly, trust me when I say all is not lost. For now, we need to meet the undeniable pull of gravity halfway and keep our feet on the ground.

Next time you set up for your hang, simply keep your feet on the floor and let your bodyweight sink down so that your knees are a little bent. Let your arms straighten and feel a nice stretch down the side of your back. *Voilà* – you are in the supported hang position! If your bar is too high and your feet won't touch the ground, find yourself a bench, a box, or anything you can use to place your feet on while you dangle. The beauty of this simple tweak is that you can adjust the intensity by adjusting how much pressure you place through your feet. As you get stronger, you can start to support yourself less with your feet and more with your arms. From there you can go from both feet to one foot, on to a gradual dangle with little toe taps, until you're soaring like the glorious eagle you are.

You can set personal challenges that match your current hang-ability, such as a goal to achieve *30 seconds total on the bar*, where you spend as long as you can dead hanging with feet off the ground, followed by as long as you can with feet on the ground.

This may start as a 5-second dead hang and a 25-second supported hang, broken into 2–3 chunks with small breaks in between. Gradually you'll literally see and feel yourself get stronger as your dead hang time increases and you rely less on the support of your feet. As always, the important part of this challenge isn't where you start, but that you're challenging yourself to get better!

Hanging Hurts?

This challenge doesn't require much movement, but there are still some simple modifications you can try.

- Try the supported hang and start with your feet on the ground, as described above.
- If it's too tough on your shoulders, spend more time working on the downward dog before introducing the hang.
- Carry a heavy weight (that you feel confident with) to improve your grip.

As always, if the issue of pain persists after attempting these adaptations, speak to a medical professional, but whatever you do, don't give up hope!

Beyond the Dangle

If you're feeling particularly spicy, which I have no doubt you are, you can build on your newfound hang-ability towards, what I believe to be, one of the greatest exercises of all time – the pull up. The move requires you to seemingly defy gravity as you temporarily overcome its hold by pulling yourself up, from your dead hang position, before lowering yourself back down. This exercise is an incredible way of challenging the strength in your back and arm muscles and while this is quite the jump from our initial hanging exploits, it's a challenge that is absolutely worth pursuing. If you're unsure how to go from hanging to pulling yourself up, here's a couple of things you can try.

1. Negative Pull ups

Instead of dangling down low with your arms fully stretched, for this variation you need to start at the top. Either start on a box or jump up so that your chin is above the bar, with the bar close to your chest (or as close as you can manage) and lower yourself down as slowly and in as controlled a manner as you possibly can. This time spent under tension on the lowering portion of the movement (also known as the eccentric if you remember from earlier) will go a long way for building strength to help you get up over the bar from our hang. Build up to 5 negative pull ups, each rep lasting at least 5 seconds from top to bottom. Once you can nail five, with control, give a full pull up a go. If you're not quite there yet you can also try . . .

2. Assisted Pull ups

There's three ways we can add some assistance to get you up over the bar. If you're a member of a gym, you may have an assisted pull up machine; this is the simplest way of adding support to your pull ups, allowing you to practise and build strength, over time reducing the support until you're ready to ride solo. If you don't have access to an assisted machine, we can simply loop a resistance band over our bar and loop it over our knee or foot. This stretchy band will work similarly to the assisted machine by giving you a boost, helping you practise the movement and build strength. Finally, if you don't have access to a band, nor machine, you can simply jump up to the bar and lower yourself down with control, like the negative pull up example above. Only as you get stronger, jump with less vigour, meaning you're using your arms more to pull, rather than legs to push. If your bar is a tad out of reach for a jump, add a box or a bench to boost you up. If you're unsure what any of these methods look like in practice and need a visual aid, search 'assisted pull ups' on YouTube: there are hundreds of demos you can work through to find what suits your set up best.

Either way, working from your hang towards a full-blown pull up is one of the most satisfying physical pursuits I've worked through with my clients and an amazing testament to your strength and ability to control and manoeuvre your own body-weight. If you're looking for an upper body fitness goal to strive for, look no further than the pull up.

Sit Down, Stand Up:
The Sit and Rise Test

Ideal for: All-round Lower Body Mobility

We're about to take it down to the floor and straight back up again with this incredible movement challenge that puts your whole-body mobility to the test. This multi-layered number requires a mixture of lower body flexibility, strength and balance as you attempt to lower yourself down to the ground and up again, hands free. If you're a little nervous about falling while doing this, set yourself up next to your sofa (or something soft) that you can use for support or as a little safety net – we're trying to improve your mobility here, not hurt you!

CHALLENGE ONE: SIT AND RISE TEST

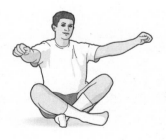

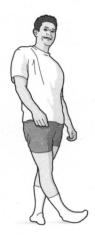

I'll say it one more time (because it's the last challenge) . . . Make sure you WHIP OUT YOUR CAMERA and record yourself!

Start standing, with your legs crossed one in front of the other, then lower yourself down to the floor in as controlled a manner as possible, until you're sitting cross-legged. Once you're down, your job is to push yourself back up to standing, using as little support from other parts of your body as possible.

TAKE NOTE

- Rate the difficulty 1–10.
- Can you sit down and stand up, hands free?
- How many times did use your hands, elbows or knees for support?
- Are you able to sit cross-legged?
- Any issues? If so, where? Pay attention to how your body feels when you're in this position and note exactly where it feels tight or 'not quite right' – the more detail the merrier.

You may well have seen or tried this challenge before. It's done the rounds on social media and rightfully so, as it's a corker of a move for testing and building your movement ability. The buzz all started with a study published in 2014 by a group of researchers in Brazil,[1] keen to explore links between the ability to move and how long you'll live. The test challenged people to perform this 'sit and rise' test, where participants were asked to lower themselves down to the floor and stand up again, using the minimum support they perceived necessary, without worrying about the speed of the movement, and then the movement was scored out of ten. Sitting down was worth five points, standing up another five, with a point deducted for each time someone used a body part to support themselves, and 0.5 points deducted for any wobbles.

The study looked at 2002 people between 51 and 80 years old and they were all asked to repeat the challenge a few times and recorded their best attempt, so if it felt a bit clunky the first time, they had the chance to give it another whirl and rescore their efforts – something which is totally open to you too as you try this move on for size. Hopefully you'll see an improvement in score immediately, or a smoother transition from standing to floor and back with just a few attempts (our brain is amazing at learning quickly!). Six years after the initial test, researchers followed up with the participants to assess their health outcomes. What is most interesting for us is that the study found that those with a lower score on the sit and rise test (0–3) had a 5–6 times higher risk of all-cause mortality than those with a higher score (8–10), with every point increase leading to a 21 per cent reduction in risk of death.

What Does This Mean?

If you can't get up and down from the floor without using your hands, your sand-timer of life isn't at its last grain. And if you bounced up and down buoyantly then I'm afraid you are no less impervious to freak accidents of life. This survival business is a bit more complicated than that. However, a higher score is reflective of a strong capacity to perform a wide variety of daily life tasks which help maintain independence, whether it's literally getting up off the floor, picking something up or getting in and out of the shower easily.

Although you won't spontaneously combust if you can't 'sit and rise' with finesse, it's worth practising. One thing I can say for sure: the longer you maintain your physical independence, the longer you can keep your heart working, and the longer you're likely to live – and the more likely those years will be a little happier, too.

So How Do I Get Better?

Aha! Wonderful question. I was hoping you'd ask. The majority of exercises sprinkled through this movement challenge series will help – especially those that involve lower body strength, flexibility, balance and stability, such as the balance, the hinge, the squat, the split squat, the 90 90 and the world's greatest stretch, the bounce. By practising these moves regularly, you will magically find that your ability to sit and rise will get better and better.

If you really want to get better at sitting down and standing up from the floor, with as little support as possible, practise doing it! To begin with you might need to rely heavily on support from your hands and knees and break the movement into stages. If you can't get up and down cross-legged, it doesn't mean practising isn't valid, it absolutely is. Use whatever technique feels intuitive for you and allows you to get up and down. Using your hands and knees will still allow you to improve, and as you get stronger you can rely on them less and less. You'd be amazed at how quickly you improve at something when you practise regularly. If you find yourself a little shaky and wobbly at the start, don't be put off! The harder you find this challenge, the more you have to benefit from practising.

Movement Challenge Summary

Oi oi! You've only gone and done it! You've made it through the movement challenges, so well done for working your way to this side of the book. I hope you've learned a thing or two about your body while getting your wiggle on, and found a few movements that hit the mobility spot. But before you put your mobility crown and gown on, I wanted to check in and help you take everything you've learned to the next level: weaving movement into your everyday life, for the rest of it.

In this section we're going to look at how to put the moves you've practised into a programme that suits your real-life schedule in order to build habits that stick. First, let's dive into a little summary of a few things you hopefully learned throughout the challenges.

These challenges were designed to do three things.

1. Explore your movement capabilities and limitations, ideally through a lens of curiosity rather than judgement.
2. Learn a bunch of moves that are pretty useful for a functioning, mobile human, and identify what the ability to do them tells you about your body.
3. Improve your bodily awareness and communication.

Hopefully you soared through them like an eagle, thinking 'Challenge? What do you mean, challenge?!' Nothing would make me happier than to hear that you breezed through these moves and proved to yourself that you've got a great foothold in this mobility game. However, it's likely there were at least a few moves that you didn't so much glide as clunk through. In those instances, if you found yourself wondering 'What's wrong with me?', the answer is: *nothing.* You don't become morally superior just because you've got a sexy squat (even if the fitness world seems to be telling you that), nor will you cease to exist if you can't touch your toes. You should never be embarrassed for not being able to do something; instead you should feel proud for trying in the first place. There is only one way to get better, and that is to practise. So don't shy away from the struggle – embrace it!

When it comes to exercise or movement in general, most of us will tend to stick to what we're good at, because we're good at it and being good at something makes us feel nice and fluffy. While this is great for honing our strengths, it means our not-so-strong bits are left even further behind, and when it comes to general mobility, it's nice to have a range of movement ability across the board. So, if you find yourself tempted to avoid the movements you struggle with the most, know that I'll be watching . . . I won't really, because that's really creepy. But please take this as a sign to give yourself a break about sucking at something.

The vast majority of us suck at something. Personally, anything that involves shoulder stability is my kryptonite – from downward doggies to push ups, side planks and tabletops. As soon as my shoulders are required to stay still under load, they threaten me with more wobbles than a jelly in an earthquake. You'll be amazed at how quickly you can improve if you're willing to ride through the initial difficult bits and stick at it. While my shoulders still like to have my pants down every now and again, after years of work, I no longer worry about my shoulder dislocating when pulling my duvet off my bed in the morning, and I've learned a hell of a lot about my body along the way.

Struggle is an opportunity for improvement, not a sign of failure.

Your Start Point

Whatever rating you gave these challenges, alongside the photos and videos you recorded of your wiggles, this is your start point! File 'em away somewhere, so you can refer back to them down the line. I'd recommend retesting every 4–6 weeks (or whenever you like, really) with new pictures, videos and the 1–10 scoring system to compare and see how you've improved.

You likely won't notice much difference practising these movements week to week, but when you whip out the retests and look at them side by side, this is where you'll notice the most progress versus when you first started. And this will earn you a surge of dopamine through your veins, which will in turn help keep you motivated. This is why the test-retest system is so saucy – it helps keep you going while showing you the fruits of your labour!

Stiffness Spectrum

By this point, it won't come as a shock when I say we're all wired to have different levels of bendiness. Some of you will be able to fold in half like a wallet, while others will feel as though your muscles are made of concrete. Again, this is a product of what yo mumma gave ya (genetics) and how much you've trained your flexibility thus far in life. This 'natural ability' applies to all components of mobility, not just flexibility, and they can all be improved. But when it comes to improving your mobility, I believe your baseline flexibility plays an important role in shaping how you should approach your training.

We all sit somewhere between a Bendy Wendy and a Big Stiff on this made-up stiffness spectrum, and even without lifting a finger or attempting any of these challenges, I'm sure you know which end of the spectrum you fall closer to. Having this awareness and understanding about your body is important because if you are on the bendier side, you may have to train a little differently than if you're on the stiffer side.

The Life of a Big Stiff

The issue with stiffness is how limited movement in one part of the body can have a knock-on effect on another. As our body moves as one big chain, if we have a particularly stiff muscle or joint, the body will compensate by finding movement elsewhere. For example, if our ankle is limited in flexibility, this might increase the forces on our knee when we walk down the stairs. If these forces exceed a joint's tolerance, over time it may cause discomfort or lead to injury. But I must stress that damage is not guaranteed just because you're on the stiffer side, but it may mean that moving freely and easily can be more difficult than it needs to be. So, when it comes to my Big Stiffs, the main focus is to get bendier and stronger. We can do this through a process of 'lengthen and strengthen', where we choose exercises that mobilise our muscles and joints. These exercises warm up the target tissue and allow us to move over larger ranges of motion. We then follow these movements with exercises that strengthen the new range of motion. While prioritising moves that stretch our stiff bits, we then pivot and add load, in the form of our bodyweight or by adding weight into the equation such as machines in the gym or free weights. By combining pauses and holds in these stretched positions, we gradually improve our strength and flexibility *at the same time*.

This two-pronged lengthen and strengthen approach helps make sure we don't just become a floppy noodle. Although it may seem simple on paper, that doesn't mean change necessarily will come easy. Changing your body's stiffness takes time and consistency, but knowing how to approach your training is half the battle. If you're a Big Stiff, you likely struggled most on exercises like the deep squat, 90 90, world's greatest stretch, shoulder dislocates, and scratch test. Basically, anything that involves flexibility.

If you're keen on working towards becoming a Medium or Mini Stiff, or maybe even a Bendy Wendy, changing your body will take time, so consistency is key. While the moves in this book certainly aren't the be all and end all for improving your flexibility and general mobility, these exercises are a brilliant place to start to get your foothold on improving your all-round flexibility, with the added benefit that you can do most of them with little more than your own body. So, there's no reason not to, aye? My advice is to look back through the movement challenges, identify something that you want to improve and challenge yourself to practise at least 2–3 times a week, with intention and intensity, and munch extra movement minutes in the form of mobility snacks wherever you can. Soon enough you *will* see improvements in how you move, specifically by shaking some of the stiffness.

The Bendy Wendy Way

However, if you're more on the Bendy Wendy side without any prior training, chances are you're already flopping around like cooked spaghetti and potentially don't need to work on your flexibility. Instead, your area of improvement is gaining control of your flexibility by focusing on strength and stability across your already extreme range of motion. You've probably heard the term 'hypermobility' being thrown round, a condition which causes individuals' joints to move beyond normal limits.

Roughly between 10 and 25 per cent of people are hyper-mobile,[1] varying from slightly more bendy than normal to more severe conditions such as Ehlers-Danlos Syndrome (EDS). An excessive range of motion can often come with complaints of longstanding pain, and it's common to experience a sensation of stiffness and a feeling of having unstable or vulnerable joints, despite appearing to move well, as well as being at greater risk of partial and full dislocations.[2] If you still feel stiff, despite being flexible, and find it almost impossible to 'hit the spot' when you stretch, it's likely you fall somewhere into this hypermobile bracket. If you're a Bendy Wendy, you will have likely struggled more with the balance challenges, such as the single leg Romanian deadlift, or strength and stability challenges like the side plank, downward dog, tabletop and Bulgarian split squat, for example.

Not everyone on the bendier side will be hypermobile, but if you're screaming 'This is me!' right now, please know that all hope is not lost. While I can't promise an exact recipe to get you out of pain, I can promise you'll benefit a huge amount from focusing on training your strength. This may involve the exercises in this book, but any form of resistance training, such as lifting weights, that develops your strength will help, just make sure you consult with a medical professional before flinging yourself at anything. Whatever you choose, the important thing is to focus on developing strength and control across your joints range of motion, rather than avoiding movement altogether, which will only lead to your body getting weaker and likely cause more issues down the line. After over 15 dislocations to my shoulder

(I wish that was an exaggeration), I can speak from experience when I say that avoiding an area that feels vulnerable will only make the problem worse. My job is to make those areas stronger and to help you build confidence in your body's ability to move through repetitions. Practice makes progress.

When moving through exercises, instead of going as far as you can, pushing to your end range of motion in search of a stretch which you might not find, I always encourage my hypermobile honeys to move slowly and not to push excessively far. This will help develop better awareness and control over your wild range of motion and identify exactly what feels vulnerable or unstable, while always maintaining control. Stop just short of your max range, where you still feel in control, and look to load this position, either by holding it for time, actively tensing the target muscles and squeezing them hard, or introducing some light weight.

This is one way to develop strength in your more compromised areas. Another tool that will be your friend is isometrics. This is a fancy way of saying 'holds' – the static freezes we dabbled in during the side plank and hangs. Adding these holds or pauses in a variety of positions across movements is a sensational way to build strength in the muscles and joints without exposing them to that feeling of instability.

While hypermobility may feel like a 'weakness' at times, for some it has the potential to be your 'mobility superpower', when harnessed with strength and control, especially if you have hopes and dreams of being a contortionist.

How Do I Know if I'm Hypermobile?

This simple self-reporting questionnaire was created to help you work it out.

- Can you now [or could you ever] place your hands flat on the floor without bending your knees?
- Can you now [or could you ever] bend your thumb to touch your forearm?
- As a child, did you amuse your friends by contorting your body into strange shapes, or could you do the splits?
- As a child or teenager, did your kneecap or shoulder dislocate on more than one occasion?
- Do you consider yourself 'double-jointed'?

Answering yes to two or more of these questions suggests hypermobility with around 84 per cent accuracy,[3] and if you want to dig a little deeper you can search the 'Beighton score', which tests your range of motion across five different manoeuvres. Both assessments have their limitations, as they only test a small number of joints, and it's either a 'yes' or 'no' rather than identifying any degree of hypermobility, but it's a starting point.

You may also find that, like myself, you have hypermobility in some joints but not all. Personally, my shoulders are like cheese strings, wobbling around all over the place, whereas my hips are far less flexy in comparison. You know your body best, and you'll get to know what it needs the more you explore and play around.

Regardless of where you find yourself on the stiffness spectrum, the aim is to work towards a body that's capable of taking its joints through their designed ranges of motion, with control, strength and stability. That is truly what will help us manoeuvre through life.

Perfect Posture

You're sat like a prawn right now, aren't you? Curled over this book like a crunchy crustacean, right? Before you freak out and sit bolt upright as if you've been caught doing something you shouldn't, chill your beans and relax. One of the questions I get asked most often is 'How can I improve my posture?' and as someone who has spent a lot of time calling everyone on the internet prawns for looking like one while they hunch over their desk (myself included), it's only fair we dedicate a chapter to our old pal, posture. Below, we're going to talk about why 'sit up straight' may not be such great advice after all, and why comfort is key to perfecting your posture.

If I asked you to show me 'bad' posture, I bet you'd fold forwards and prawn (I know this isn't a verb – *yet* – but I'm hoping if I use it enough, I can make it stick). I'm talking about rounding your shoulders, pushing your head forwards and letting your arms slump by your side. In order words, slouching. Earlier, I used the term 'kyphosis' to describe this prawn-like posture. If I asked you to assume a 'good' posture, I bet you'd stand, or sit up straight, with your head held high, shoulders pinned down and back, with your chest out to the world, as if you were standing to attention. The idea of 'good' and 'bad' posture is ingrained in us at a societal level and we've all likely had someone at some point, whether it was a teacher, coach or family member, nag at us to sit up straight, as if it's impossible to listen or function as a human the moment you start slouching. But is there really such a thing as 'good' or 'bad' posture, and does it have the ability to predict anything about our health outcomes?

'Bad' posture has consistently been linked with back pain,[1] and labels such as 'upper and lower cross syndrome', 'kyphosis', 'lordosis', 'scoliosis', 'anterior pelvic tilt' and 'text neck' get thrown around as explanations for one of the most common causes of disability in humans: lower back pain.[2] Back pain is, without a doubt, one of the most debilitating things I've ever experienced. For me, it started when I was 15, and has plagued me on and off throughout my twenties, and even now I find myself experiencing flare-ups from time to time, especially when I push my stress levels too far. In 2020 there were approximately 619 million cases of lower back pain, globally.[3] That's one hell of a lot of back pain around the world and chances are it has, or will, afflict you at some point, too. A survey of 2,184 people between the ages 20–69 found that over 84 per cent of people asked had experienced lower back pain at some point in their life.[4] Considering this doesn't account for those older than 69, it may be safe to assume that prevalence of lower back pain is even higher, and for a long time it's been believed to be associated with poor posture. But is our prawn-like behaviour really to blame?

First off the bat, the good news is that research seems to suggest that for most of us, recovery from lower back pain is pretty quick, where the majority of people (70 per cent in this study) recover after just one week and 90 per cent in six weeks.[5] So, if you're currently in the back pain camp, the prognosis is in your favour, but if you are concerned about your posture, hopefully I can put your mind at ease.

The issue with the terms 'good' and 'bad' when it comes to talking about posture is that, like most things in life, it's not as black and white as simply categorising any one position as good and another as bad. I'm going to try my best to change your perspective on how you view your posture and how to best take care of that saucy spine of yours, by moving away from this binary view of 'good' and 'bad' and encouraging you to embrace the grey.

What does the science say? This meta-analysis (remember the big study of studies?) looked at 43 different research papers analysing lumbo-pelvic kinematics, which is just a fancy way of saying lower back and hip movement and positions, in people with and without back pain. They found no difference in lower back curvature (lordosis angle) or standing pelvis position (pelvic tilt angle)[6], meaning if you have an anterior or posterior pelvic tilt and a butt that sticks out, you probably shouldn't worry about it and it's unlikely to be the reason for back pain. These findings are consistently echoed elsewhere with another meta-analysis (this one looking at another 54 studies), which found no association between spinal posture and pain.[7] The reality is none of us have just 'one' posture. Our spine is made up of 33 individual bones connected by 'discs' of cartilage to form joints, which allow us to assume a variety of positions depending on the demands of our environment. Whether we're sitting, standing or lying down, the position we find ourselves in is mostly a subconscious choice and a result of both our genetics, which make up the structure of our body, and whatever we find most comfortable at that moment in time. This, of course, is also based on whatever it is we're doing, but no matter what that is, we're not fixed into any ideal position or posture. You can easily make changes to your posture just by changing position.

Hunching over like a prawn may not be the sexiest position I'll ever assume (although that's up for debate), but I think we can both agree it's a lot comfier than trying to sit up straight all day. If you don't believe me, try sitting bolt upright as you read the rest of this chapter and see how you feel afterwards. It's bloody tiring! But don't just take my word for it. A recent study followed

686 people over five years and compared their postures. When it came to the results, the researchers found that those who slumped had a *lower* risk of persistent neck pain compared to those that consistently held more upright postures.[8]

I think we can draw a lesson or two here from smiling. There's nothing nicer than seeing someone smile; it's infectious and has a beautiful ability to rub off on us. It also subconsciously makes somebody appear more attractive – a lot like standing up straight, tall and proud. But if you spent all day smiling, your face and jaw would be knackered by the end of it, and you'd probably look a bit creepy after a while too. If you try to stay this rigid all the time, in smile or posture, it's no surprise that things start to hurt after a while.

Smiling is reflective of our mood, and so is posture.[9] A good test for this is if I asked you to draw a sad person, it's likely you'd depict a big ol' slouch alongside a frown, whereas if I asked you to draw a happy person, you'd likely imagine someone standing tall, head high, chest to the world (don't worry, you don't have to actually draw – I can't either).

Standing up straight may be more aesthetically pleasing and something we subconsciously associate with status and wellbeing, but it doesn't automatically improve your spinal health. What's more, attempting to maintain a rigid upright posture all day may do more harm than good, especially if it comes at the cost of comfort. On the other hand, prawning may not look as appealing, but it shouldn't be feared – it's comfy, after all. Sitting too still or rigidly for a long time is more likely to be a problem for most people than slouching.

To say that any one position is better than another as a rule of thumb is naive when we consider the variety of bodies across the eight billion of us on the planet. What each person finds comfy may look radically different. So, when it comes to our health, it's about time we scrapped this black and white idea of 'postural perfection' and embraced the grey. Instead of good and bad posture, the question you should be asking yourself is 'when did I last *change* my posture, and am I comfortable?' In other words, be the prawn, if you want – just don't spend your whole life like it. No one position is automatically better than another, and your spine is robust and adaptable, but in order to keep it that way, you need to move it – often.

So, what's the beef with staying still all day? Well, I like to think of our body like a big pump, and every time we move, it pumps liquids such as blood and synovial fluid (aka joint lube) *filled* with nutrients and goodness all around the bod. But when we stay still for long periods of time, this fluid becomes stagnant and leached of fresh metabolites. This is one of the major reasons that movement is so important. It's also why when it comes to posture: your best posture is your next posture.

Your Best Posture is Your Next Posture

So how often should you change places and position? In the spirit of embracing the grey, the answer I'm going to give you is annoyingly vague: 'move as much as possible'. If it helps to have something specific, aim for every 20–30 minutes, but don't get too hung up on the specifics. It may help to set regular reminders to shuffle position, and slap reminders on your laptop or phone to nudge you every now and again. Or if you find yourself jumping from call to call, challenge yourself to take each one in a different position to keep your movement flowing. Whether that be a different workstation at home or at work, or challenging yourself to move through a few exercises in this book while you work, like the 90 90, the squat or the elephant walks. In the same breath, I also want to reassure you that sitting still for longer than 30 minutes won't automatically do damage, and it certainly won't kill you – you're a lot more robust than that. There will be times you're wired to your desk to meet a deadline, stuck on a long-haul flight or on a long car journey, and there'll be very little you can do about it. Just try to move and wiggle as often as you can, and, where possible, avoid sitting still for ridiculously long periods of time.

Speaking of which, I think it's about time you CHANGE PLACES, don't you? This is my little nudge to stand up, have a wiggle, and sit in a different place or position if you can. Maybe change your seat or cross your legs the other way. Whatever you do, have a little shuffle – this is part of what taking care of your posture should look like.

If you're trying to impress in a job interview, it's probably worthwhile sitting up straight and smiling, but you don't need to spend your whole life like that. There's nothing wrong with a little prawning.

So instead of asking 'How can I improve my posture?', if you want to be a loving servant to your spine, the better questions to ask are 'Am I comfy?' and 'Am I changing position regularly enough?'

Remember: *your best posture is your next posture.*

Building the Habit

It's all well and good giving you a load of mobility moves and theories, but I want this stuff to stick with you for life, like a tattoo you wear with pride. The dream is for movement to become so embedded in your world that, without even thinking about it, you're wiggling left, right and centre at every opportunity. There is no change without change, so I wanted to whizz through some of my best habit-moulding strategies to help you and movement become two peas in a pod.

The aim of this section is to use some of my top tips and tricks to make movement a more consistent feature in your life, via:

1. Dedicated workouts
2. Wiggles throughout the day

Dedicated Workouts

Your Buffer Zone

When it comes to the 'ideal' amount of exercise in a week, we're not looking for the optimal amount to get the best results. I know that might sound a bit backwards, but we're looking for the amount that you can genuinely stick to. *That* is the ideal amount of exercise. No matter how much or how little that is, your best results will come from what you do consistently over a long period of time. There's no point looking for the 'ideal' amount if it drives you to throw in the towel after the first week, ya feel me?

Here are some questions to get you thinking about what the ideal amount might look like to you. Grab a pen and paper, or scribble these down in the notes of your phone – it's time to do some planning!

- In an ideal world, how many workouts would you like to do each week?
- What is the maximum amount of time you can dedicate to these workouts?

Whatever you've scribbled down will be your goal for the week ahead. But before you skip into the sunset, revelling in your currently motivated state and determined to dominate your workouts this week, I need you to answer one more question.

- What's the absolute minimum number of workouts you will 100 per cent commit to this week, regardless of what is going on in your world?

If you have no idea where to start, a great aim is three workouts per week, with an absolute minimum non-negotiable (unless your legs fall off) of one. This is a sensational start point if the idea of habitual exercise feels a little foreign, or you've struggled to stick to a workout programme in the past.

In case you're thinking, 'But Adam, I've committed to the first goal, why would I even entertain an amount lower than that?' Well, here's the kicker. If we want this habit to stick, we need a sprinkle of honesty. I'd absolutely love you to smash every workout every week without fail, but the motivated human writing these goals can't speak for the future you. Now-you and future-you are two different people, and no matter how much you plan, promise or prioritise your workouts, there will come a time when the shit hits the fan – when emergency strikes and your cat swallows an entire cotton bud (yes, I'm speaking from experience), you simply get ill, or you have to work late and cannot be bothered to do a workout after a long day of life. When it comes to building an exercise habit, you need to set yourself up to win. If you say you're going to do three workouts a week, but end up doing two, you're likely going to feel that you've failed – unnecessarily, may I add.

But by having the foresight to give yourself a buffer to say 'Not today, world', then if, for whatever reason, you only get one workout done that week, you're much more likely to pat yourself on the back because you did what you said you were going to do, helping you internalise doing your workout as a good thing, rather than this idea that missing a workout is a failure.

This tiny shift in perspective goes a long way in shaping a positive perception of exercise. If you constantly say you're going to do something but don't, you're fooling yourself, and no one wants to be fooled. Instead, bring the goalposts closer and smash them. You'll be surprised how good it feels when you start exceeding your expectations, rather than always falling short of them.

One workout a week might not feel like much, but it's still 52 in a year. I guarantee if you do anything 52 times in a year, you'll get better at it. Would I like you to work out more than once a week? Sure. Multiple weekly workouts will expedite your health endeavours massively. But let's be real, who's going to get better results, somebody who does 52 workouts in a year, or someone who does 10 in two weeks and gives up?

Set ambitious goals to strive for, but cushion them with realistic, non-negotiable targets and make sure you hit them as often as possible. Anything over these 'non-negotiables' is an added bonus. This buffer zone is a really powerful tool to help you shift from an 'all or nothing' mindset towards a 'something is always better than nothing' approach.

Always remember that your progress won't be made or broken by one missed workout. Your success is a product of your choices over a long period of time – that's what really matters. The only way you fail this mobility game is if you give up completely.

When it comes to achieving the commendable action of dedicated exercise sessions, it helps to have a programme to follow, so here's some I made earlier!

I've taken all the exercises from the movement challenge series and slipped them into a few easy-to-follow sequences that you can squeeze into your life, based on the time you have available, for true mobility world domination.

Try not to overcomplicate things. Choose one of the plans below and see if it works for you. If not, give a different one a bash. The aim of these programmes is to show that there are plenty of ways to break up these workouts while still giving each exercise a decent run through. Some require fewer days but more time, others more days but less time. You may find that some weeks the All in One approach works best, while other weeks you need Little by Little. The only person who knows what's best for you is you. All I care about is that you're doing something, not how you choose to do it. The best programme is the one that fits your life, that you can genuinely stick to.

1. **All in One** (1–4 days per week) With this format, we're busting out the whole shebang at once, rolling our way through one round of 20+ moves. This is perfect for people who have fewer days to commit to their mobility training in a week and like getting it all done in one go. I'd recommend starting with this format to get the hang of each move, but of course, you know your schedule and your body best.

EXERCISE	SETS AND REPS
Bounce	1 × 1 Min
90 90 Transitions	1 × 10 / Side
Glute Bridge	1 × 10
Couch Stretch	1 × 30s / Side
World's Greatest Stretch	1 × 10 / Side
Split Squat	1 × 10 / Side
Elephant Walk	1 × 10 / Side
Single Leg RDL (Hinge)	1 × 10 / Side
Squat	1 × 10
Deep Squat Hold	1 × 30s
Side Plank Lift	1 × 10 / Side
Side Plank Hold	1 × 30s / Side
Shoulder Dislocates	1 × 10
Hands Behind Your Back Floss	1 × 10 / Side
Downward Dog	1 × 10
Downward Dog Hold	1 × 30s
Cobra Push Up	1 × 10
Cobra Hold	1 × 30s
Prone Press	1 × 10
Push Up	1 × 10
Tabletop Lift	1 × 10
Bonus: Hang	1 × Max time

Complete the exercises back-to-back, one after another, with as much or as little rest as you need. The workout will take roughly 25–45 minutes, depending on how familiar you are with the exercises and how much rest time you take. To begin, you'll want to block out a bit of extra time to get familiar with the exercises and take rest breaks.

To get the best of this format, I'd aim to do this workout around 1–4 times a week, with a rest day between each session. Chances are you'll feel a bit stiff and sore in the beginning, especially if you've never done this before or if the exercises are new. It's worth remembering that you don't need to do this every day to benefit.

You'll see the best results if you practice 3–4 times a week, with sufficient intensity, but that doesn't mean you won't benefit from doing the exercises only once or twice, because something is always better than nothing. Even if it's only once a week to begin with, that's still a step in the right direction. Alternatively, if you feel great and want to incorporate this routine as a daily practise, you can too. You're the boss of you after all, just listen to your body and remember that more isn't always merrier, we need stress plus *rest* to grow.

Example week:

> Monday: All in One
> Tuesday: Go for a walk
> Wednesday: All in One
> Thursday: Walk and gentle practice (e.g. 90 90 and deep squat)
> Friday: All in One
> Saturday: Rest
> Sunday: Gentle skill practice, such as balance, single leg
>   RDL and bounce

2. **Up and Down** (2–6 days per week) This method splits the exercises across two days, one focusing above the waist, the other below. This breaks the programme into smaller chunks across more days of the week, but with the option to repeat each exercise a couple of times for a little more practice. This is perfect for somebody who already goes to the gym and wants to work more mobility-specific training around their schedule.

229

LOWER BODY DAY

EXERCISE	SETS AND REPS
1A – Bounce	2 × 1 Min
1B – 90 90 Transitions	2 × 15 / Side
2A – Glute Bridge	2 × 15 / Side
2B – World's Greatest Stretch	2 × 10
3A – Elephant Walk	2 × 15 / Side
3B – Couch Stretch	2 × 30s / Side
4A – Split Squat	2 × 10 / Side
4B – Single Leg RDL (Hinge)	2 × 10 / Side
5A – Squat	2 × 10
5B – Deep Squat Hold	2 × 30s
6A – Side Plank Lift	2 × 10 / Side
6B – Side Plank Hold	2 × 30s / Side

UPPER BODY DAY

1A – Jefferson Curl	2 × 10
1B – Shoulder Dislocates	2 × 10
1C – Towel Floss	2 × 10 / Side
2A – Downward Dog Transition	2 × 10
2B – Downward Dog Hold	2 × 30s
3A – Cobra Push Up	2 × 10
3B – Cobra Hold	2 × 30s
4A – Prone Press	2 × 10
4B – Push Up	2 × 10
5A – Tabletop Lift	2 × 10
5B – Tabletop Hold	2 × 30s
Bonus: Hang	2 × Max time

Here, exercises are numbered and lettered e.g. 1A, 1B and 1C to group them into areas of focus. Complete all the exercises with the same number back-to-back before moving on to the next. Exercises are to be repeated twice, so do 10 reps of exercise A, 10 reps of exercise B, and then go back to A for another round. Take as much or as little rest as you need. The workout will take roughly 20–30 minutes, again depending on how familiar you are with the movements and how much rest you take in between.

With this up and down format, you can work out on back-to-back days. I'd recommend doing two days on, one day off to get the best out of this format.

Example week:

Monday: Lower
Tuesday: Upper
Wednesday: Rest
Thursday: Lower
Friday: Upper
Saturday: Rest
Sunday: Rest

3. **Little by Little** Doing something almost every day of the week in 10–15-minute chunks. This is for my pals that just don't have the time and/or inclination to commit to long workouts, but still know they've got to move. This is a great doorway to making mobility training more accessible and building up to bigger workouts over time.

DAY 1

1A – Bounce	3 x 1 Min
1B – Single Leg Balance	3 x 30s / Side
1C – Hang	3 x Max time

DAY 2

1A – 90 90 Transitions	3 × 15
1B – World's Greatest Stretch	3 × 10 / Side
2A – Squat	3 × 15
2B – Deep Squat Hold	3 × 30s

DAY 3

1A – Shoulder Dislocates	1 × 20
2A – Downward Dog Transitions	3 × 15
2B – Downward Dog Holds	3 × 30s
3A – Cobra Push Up	3 × 15
3B – Cobra Hold	3 × 30s

DAY 4

1A – Elephant Walk	2 × 15 / Side
1B – Couch Stretch	2 × 30s / Side
2A – Single Leg Glute Bridge	3 × 15 / Side
2B – Split Squat	3 × 10 / Side
3A – Single Leg Romanian Deadlift	3 × 10 / Side

DAY 5

1A – Hands Behind Back Floss	1 × 10 / Side
2A – Prone W Press	3 × 20
2B – Push Up	3 × 20

DAY 6

1A – Tabletop Lift	3 × 10
1B – Tabletop Hold	3 × 30s
2A – Side Plank Lift	3 × 10
2B – Side Plank Hold	3 × 30s

Notes About the Programme

The sets, repetitions and times in these programmes are just targets. Work at a level that challenges you but doesn't feel overwhelming – there's nothing special about hitting 10 reps, it's just an aim. If any of the exercises feel impossible, choose an easier version of the move from the challenges in this book. Conversely, if an exercise feels too easy, you can progress onto a harder variation. I know I waffle a lot about not rushing and taking it at your own pace, but I really do mean it. This ain't a race. If you can't make it to 10 reps with ease, focus on 'mastering' the movement rather than the numbers. Move super slow and add pauses. Whatever you do, take your time. I'd much rather you focus on doing one good-quality rep than try to smash through 10 reps of each exercise.

The purpose of these programmes is to foster confidence and competence with each movement by building control. The idea is that the moves become so easy over time that they no longer feel like exercise.

Making Progress

When it comes to getting fitter there's a fundamental principle we need to consider known as 'progressive overload'. This is a spicy way of saying: in order to grow, you need to continually challenge yourself. If you want to improve your strength, flexibility, stamina or any other area of your fitness, we need to challenge you sufficiently to stimulate change in your body. In order to keep progressing it means that we need to keep increasing the amount of challenge we expose our body to. There are *loads* of ways we can do this, but here's a few to add to your tool belt.

1. Increase the number of reps performed
2. Increase the number of sets performed
3. Increase the frequency of sessions
4. Reduce rest in between exercises
5. Increase range of motion of an exercise
6. Slow down the movement, add pauses and increase time under tension
7. Add external load, such as resistance bands or weights to increase challenge
8. Progress on to a more challenging variation of an exercise

While this isn't an exhaustive list of all ways to progressively overload your training, these tools should help you sprinkle some spice into your training, once you feel things get a little too easy, to ensure that you keep growing.

Tracking Progress

There are loads of ways you can track progress in your mobility as you get deeper into the programmes. The main improvements you'll see will come from retesting the challenges every 4–6 weeks, but don't feel you have to stick to these religiously. Just WHIP OUT YOUR CAMERA and retest if you feel like you're making progress and want to check.

What to look for:

- Bendier: you're able to move across a larger range of motion.
- More stable: you visually wobble a lot less.
- Better coordination: you're more in control of the movement and look more fluid.
- Stronger: you hold positions for longer, probably less grimacing too.

Don't just rely on visual feedback. Pay attention to what you *feel:*

- Stronger: the exercises feel easier. You can complete more reps, more sets, and hold positions for longer, without getting tired as quickly.
- Stability: you feel less wobbly.
- Relaxed: you feel more relaxed and in control of your breath as you move. You can move slower, and you feel more coordinated. Something that once took a lot of brain power and laser-focused attention doesn't take as much thought.
- Fitter: something that was once an 8/10 now feels like 6/10, and your heart isn't pounding out of your chest while you're trying do it. You're not sweating as much, or as soon into the workout.

Your progress will be unique to you, and it almost definitely won't happen in a straight line. In some sessions you'll feel like you've come on leaps and bounds; in others it may feel like you've gone backwards. But whatever happens, the most important thing is that you keep going.

Maintaining Progress

For some of us it's not always about making progress as much as it is about maintaining our ability to do the things we love. There won't always be a desire to get stronger or bendier and that's absolutely fine. In fact, if you're happy with what you can currently do that's amazing. Simply maintaining the ability to do things we need to do is an incredible goal and one that so many of us overlook. If this is you and you can already do most of what you want, the good news is that you don't need to do anything drastic, or even worry about progressively overloading your exercises, you simply need to keep doing them and exposing your body to those positions regularly. So, if the movements in this book are important to your 'why', just make sure you keep doing them a couple of times a week to keep the body ticking, and don't worry about getting too caught up in how you can continually progress. Happiness with what you have is the ultimate goal.

How to Stay Consistent with Your Workouts

Once you've figured out how many workouts you're ideally going to do, and your minimum non-negotiable commitment, it's time to plan them into your week. My maths teacher always used to say things like 'fail to prepare, prepare to fail' and 'piss poor preparation promotes piss poor performance'. As a 15-year-old who cared about anything but revising for my GCSEs, I found these sayings really annoying, but like most old adages, there's some truth there too. If you want to get your workouts done, you've got to treat them as a priority, not an afterthought. I'm not expecting you to go all militant here, but a little planning goes a long way in reducing friction between you and your workouts.

Put Your Workouts in Your Calendar

Chances are, if you book in a meeting or organise an appointment, you'd pop it in your calendar to make sure nothing else came up and clashed with it. So treat your workouts as if they were an important business meeting with the CEO (you). Before the start of each week, take five minutes and plan when and where you'll be doing your workouts and how they realistically fit into your days. If you're not working out at home, consider how long it takes you to get to and from the gym or studio, or wherever you're planning to move. Make sure you plan for the maximum number of sessions you're aiming for in a week and be specific and schedule an exact time where possible.

For me, I prefer a physical calendar. That way I can put it somewhere obvious, like on the fridge or on my desk, and I can't avoid it staring at me. I know I'm a lot less likely to ignore it than if it were on my phone or laptop. But hey, you do you.

Get Your Kit Out

Depending on when you've scheduled your workouts, make sure you've got everything you need ready to go. Lay out your workout clothes the night before, or put them in your bag to take to work with you. Set up your yoga mat and get your resistance bands out ready to roll. You're a lot more likely to get stretching if all the kit is there, staring you in the face.

This tiny bit of preparation before you go into your day will go a long way in supporting you to keep your commitment to yourself. It will also stop you getting to the end of the week and thinking, 'I said I was going to do three workouts. It's Sunday and I've done none, oops.'

Tick 'Em Off

Every time you get one of your workouts done, give yourself a big ol' tick, X, or gold star – whatever makes you feel jazzy inside! Every workout you miss, circle it. I don't know what it is about ticking something off on a calendar or a to-do list. Maybe it's reminiscent of getting a gold star at school, who knows. Either way – it feels good!

At the end of the month, look for two things:

1. Did you stick to your minimum, non-negotiable workout goal this month?

If the answer is no, shake it off and aim to be better next month. This is inevitably going to happen at some point, and if it was because of circumstances out of your control, no biggie. If it was down to poor planning or a strong case of 'can't be arsed', either reassess your non-negotiables or your planning abilities, and remember *why* you're doing this in the first place. When we miss once, we don't miss twice, so make next month your month.

If yes, well done! You've achieved the minimum you set out to. This is a big win for your accountability. If you can keep this up every single month as an *absolute minimum*, I'll bet my left ear you'll make substantial progress and be in a much better position with your mobility this time next year.

But we ain't done yet. There's levels to this consistency game, and the next thing we want to know is . . .

2. How many workouts did you total in the month versus how many you set out to do (aka your percentage consistency)?

Add up how many workouts you did over the month and divide it by the number of workouts you'd planned in total, and this will tell you your *consistency percentage*.

10 workouts completed / 12 planned workouts = 0.8 (= 80 per cent)

While you ultimately get to decide what level of consistency is a win, here's a fruity traffic light system to guide you.

>80% = Gold	You're killing this consistency game! This is really where you want to be: in a good balance between setting realistic workout frequency goals, while still allowing some flexibility for life. You're hitting 4/5 of your workouts, while allowing yourself some space to say, 'I'd rather have a beer with some mates today, I'll get at it again tomorrow.'
66–79% = Green	You're still in the sweet spot for consistency. You're smashing at least 2/3 of all your planned workouts. You could easily cruise here for the rest of your days and make incredible progress, but there's still room for improvement should you want it.
50–65% = Amber	You'll make plenty of progress at this level. But if you're consistently falling into this bracket, it's likely you're overestimating how much you can commit to in a week. You're hitting just over half of your planned workouts, which is still great, but it could be better. It might be worth going back to the drawing board and reframing your expectations, goals or planning.
<50% = Red	Tough month at the office! Things obviously haven't gone to plan, but instead of getting frustrated, it's time to look at the goals you're setting for yourself or the planning of your workouts. Either way, make it your mission to see a higher % next month!

This consistency calendar is not a must. Getting all 'maths-y' with your progress isn't for everyone. But, if you've struggled with consistency in the past, or you're new to regular exercise, this is a banging way of encouraging you to focus on the process and not just the outcome, while adding a little gamification into the mix. It's great to have some healthy competition with yourself, so aiming to beat your previous month's consistency percentage can go a long way for really firing your motivation (especially if you dangle a cute reward or two for yourself at the end).

Most people don't use this calendar forever. After 3–6 months the foundations of the workout habit are a bit more firmly laid, the rewards from your physical pursuits a little more apparent, the motivation flows a little easier and you rely less on the calendar-based feedback to give you a pat on the back. But if you want to give yourself every chance of success, committing to using a calendar for the next few months will go a hell of a long way in teaching you to plan and organise your workouts. At the same time, it will also give you the feedback and data to show you're on the right track, adding that little bit of extra accountability.

A large part of building an exercise habit is overcoming the mental barriers and realising that you don't need to be 100 per cent consistent in order to make progress. To get the highest possible degree classification at university in the UK you need to get 70 per cent. Not 100 per cent, not 90 per cent. Just 70 per cent gets you a first-class degree. Yet when it comes to building a habit around fitness, it can feel like you need to be 100 per cent perfect in order to progress. If we adopted a more consistent but flexible approach with a bit of leeway, and also rewarded ourselves for being consistent, I think most of us would find we make all the progress we want, without beating ourselves up along the way.

Le Gym

This section is for all the gym bunnies out there! Most of this book is aimed at helping us everyday humans fulfil their movement potential without needing a gym. Nevertheless, as someone who's learned to develop a love of the process and appreciation for the 'me time' that comes with going to the gym, I want to dedicate a small section of the book to ways you can approach your sessions to get as much out of your mobility mission as possible.

The gym isn't the be all and end all when it comes to health and mobility. Fundamentally, when it comes to improving your movement ability, the most important thing is working out ways you can incorporate movement into your daily life, for life. Movement that builds strength, flexibility, stamina, balance and coordination. Ideally in a form that you enjoy (or at least can tolerate and that you value). I don't believe that anybody *needs* to go to the gym in order to fulfil their mobility potential. I'm pretty sure my nan never did, but she exercised regularly, and she was still playing badminton into her eighties.

Though you certainly don't need to go to the gym to build a body that lasts, as a building designed to get you stronger and fitter, it's as convenient as it gets. So, if you have a bubbling interest I absolutely encourage you to dip your toes in, I promise it's not as scary as it seems once you know your way around, and with the right approach it can work wonders for your joint health as well as your muscles, heart and head. And there's the added bonus that you're less likely to flop on the sofa and not get up in between exercises (we've all done it).

Here are a few tips to help you get the best out of your mobility during your gym sessions.

Warm Up

If you're unsure how to warm up for your gym sessions, check out the chapter on page 271. Spending some time warming up the body is going to help limber up your muscles and joints and access a little more range of motion. This doesn't mean you have to spend 20 minutes doing mobility work before your actual workout, but spending 5–10 minutes raising your pulse and core temperature will work wonders before diving into your main exercises. My personal favourite is the 'assault' or 'air' bike. They have them in most gyms and they're a great piece of kit for getting the upper and lower body working – play around and find what you enjoy. This is also a great time to introduce a little movement variety and get your body moving in all sorts of ways that you maybe wouldn't experience in your day-to-day life.

Exercise Selection

Choosing the right exercises is key for building your mobility in the gym, but what should you be looking for? While all exercises have the potential to aid your mobility to a certain degree, simply by exposing you to movement, combining the right exercises together can have an incredible impact on your mobility potential.

Prioritise Movements That Work Ranges of Motion You Want to Improve or Maintain

If you want to improve your hamstring flexibility while training in the gym, you're going to need to choose exercises that stretch your hamstrings under load, such as a Romanian deadlift (aka your hinge – see page 79) and accumulate time in the stretched position by adding pauses. This will help improve the flexibility of the muscle in question and you can apply this concept to almost anywhere in the body (within reason) by choosing exercises that expose you to a stretch. That being said, I'd like to point out that improving range of motion doesn't always just mean jamming your joints into their end ranges of motion and chasing a stretch. For most of us, we'll benefit a lot by improving the control over the range of motion we already have. If you just want to maintain your range of motion, rather than increase it, make sure you're choosing exercises that regularly expose your body to the movement patterns you want to keep, such as those in this book. This will indicate to your brain that those movements are important and should be held on to at all costs.

Pairing Exercises Together: Lengthen and Strengthen

Lengthening and strengthening is the name of the mobility game, and this means choosing exercises that mobilise the joints and muscles we're about to use before we do our 'main exercise'. The premise is to lengthen the tissues, and then strengthen across our new range of motion.

For example, if you wanted to improve your squat depth, you might spend some time mobilising your ankles and hips before you squat, so your session might start like this:

- Warm up: 5–10-minute incline walking on a treadmill
- 3 sets of calf raises, with hip 90 90 transitions while you rest between sets to improve ankle dorsiflexion and hip internal external rotation, needed to get deep into a squat
- Then go into squats

Now that your ankles and hips have been lubed up and mobilised, you'll be able to get a little deeper into your squat and build strength across a larger range of motion (yay). Flexibility and strength at the same time – the ultimate combo.

You can apply this to any exercise by identifying which joints and muscles you're about to use in your main exercise and adding a mobility-specific move before doing so that lengthens the target tissues before you strengthen them. You don't have to do this with every exercise, but if you have a specific restriction you want to improve, lengthen and then strengthen that puppy with this approach.

Stretch During Your Rest Periods

Instead of jumping on your phone between sets, wiggle into a stretch for 30 seconds. How you choose which bit you stretch is totally up to you. If you have a stiff bit you want to attend to, this is the perfect opportunity. For me personally, the stretch I choose will depend on the exercise I'm doing. I'll either stretch the muscles I'm working or the muscles on the opposing side of the body. How do I decide which? If the main exercise I'm doing already involves a big stretch, I'll stretch the opposing, antagonist muscles. If there's not much stretch involved, I'll stretch the muscles I'm working.

Examples:

Romanian deadlift = big stretch on my hamstrings. So, while I rest, I'll stretch my hip flexors with a couch stretch or hip flexor lunge.

Chest press = Not a huge stretch on this exercise for me, so I'll stretch the pecs and shoulders while I rest.

Alternatively, you could stretch your lower body between sets on upper body days, and vice versa. If I'm honest, I really don't know which is more or *most* effective; ask me again in 20 years and maybe I'll have an answer. Either way, get productive in your rest periods and do some stretching; you'll likely get a lot more out of your workouts and won't feel guilty if you end up sacking off the stretching at the end of your session.

Research seems to indicate that stretching between sets may even enhance muscle growth, when the target muscle is stretched immediately after the last repetition for 20–30 seconds.[1] While I can't promise the effect will be massive on muscle growth, it's an amazing, time effective way of squeezing in more targeted movement minutes.

Full Range of Motion + Pauses

Choosing an exercise that works a range of motion you want to improve only works if you train the exercise across the full range of motion. While this doesn't mean pushing as far and as hard as you possibly can, if you want to improve your mobility it does mean dipping your toe into the stretch. My rule here is to go to the point you can feel the stretch and pause. Hold the position for 2–5 seconds, or roughly one big, deep breath, before pushing yourself back up again. These pauses accumulate more time in the stretch, while under extra load, which helps strengthen these positions and improve flexibility at the same time.

Get Stronger

There aren't many more beneficial things you can do for your mobility than simply getting stronger. Chances are if you're in the gym and throwing around some weights, you're well on your way, but making dedicated efforts to challenge yourself to lift more weight, gradually and steadily over time with greater control, is everything for maintaining healthy muscles as we age, and needed an honourable mention in this section.

While this isn't a totally comprehensive guide to everything you can do in the gym to improve your mobility, applying these concepts into your gym sessions will go a long way to helping you develop your flexibility and strength at the same time. Flexy and sexy – win win.

Moving More Throughout the Day

We love our mobility training sessions round here. Those dedicated windows are our meat and gravy (or meat substitute and gravy), where we really get down and dirty and spend some serious (or not so serious) one-on-one time with our body, aiming to execute our exercises to the best of our ability, hone our breath and become the mobility daddy (or mummy). But there's a lot of life lived outside of these sessions, and that means there are a lot of extra wiggles to be wiggled. Though our dedicated sessions are important, some of the greatest contributions to our mobility come from what we do throughout our day. I like to see that as the veg and potatoes, the unsung heroes of the roast dinner.

You might have realised by now that I like using basic maths to illustrate my points. Something about seeing the numbers helps me put this exercise fluff into perspective when it comes to building a body that lasts. So . . . three All in One mobility sessions (page 227) could be anywhere between one to two hours of dedicated mobility practice a week, which is an amazing start. With 168 hours in a week, assuming you're sleeping 8 hours a night, that leaves 112 waking hours. Minus the two hours a week dedicated to your training sessions, that's 1.8 per cent of your week. Our job is to fill the remaining 98.2 per cent of your week with as much wiggling as possible. Because in all honesty, if you're spending <2 per cent of your week training your mobility, but the other 98 per cent still as a statue, your body probably isn't going to feel tip top. I'm not expecting you to become a non-stop fidget, but I'm sure you and I can agree it would be a good idea to fill some downtime with a few shimmies and shakes to keep the blood pumping and the joint lube flowing.

Here are some of my top wiggle-working tips to help fill your day with movement.

Brush Your Joints:
Two Minutes of Mornin' Movin'

From day one – well, from the day we first have teeth and functioning hand-eye coordination – we're encouraged to brush our teeth, twice a day, to help keep 'em clean. I bet for most of you, the idea of brushing your teeth twice a day is almost instinctive, with little thought given to the matter. It's just something you do. Your teeth won't fall out and you won't need a filling if you don't brush them once, but forget them altogether and eventually you'll need a dentist-based intervention. Your joints are no different. I'm sure you're bored of me waffling on about joint health at this point, and I'm sure if you've made it this far then you don't need convincing, but the point I'm trying to make is that, like brushing your teeth, if you want to maintain healthy joints, it's a good idea to carve a little joint TLC into your mornings and nights.

Before or after you brush those face pegs of yours in the morning and evening, whip out your phone, set a 2-minute timer, and move. Before you ask what moves you should do, don't overthink it, just move. Not only do you have a bank of suggestions throughout this book, but you also have a body that needs exploring. Play around! This is your opportunity to throw your limbs about, ideally gently, and see how your body feels in the morning and at night. When you find a stiff bit, spend time in that position having a good ol' BREATHE!

This is your chance to build your own movement routine, filled with moves that feel good to you, and it doesn't always have to be a structured practice to help. See this as your own personal interpretive dance, your chance to contort your body in all kinds of different ways to start and end the day.

Only 2 Minutes?

Hey, a lot of magic can happen in 2 minutes. Don't knock it until you've tried it. To be honest, the 2 minutes is just to get you going, because getting started is the hardest part. You're a lot more likely to do it if it's only 2 minutes, versus 5, 10 or 15. And I know what you're like: chances are, once you're wriggling around, bouncing about your bedroom, getting all stretchy stretchy, you'll find yourself 10 minutes deep and still moving. Sneaky, aye?

Don't worry, you don't have to deceive yourself all the time. Some days you will literally only have 2 minutes, but 2 minutes twice a day is still 24 hours of wiggling in a year. That's an entire day of mobility practice in a year, just from a couple of minutes shaking your booty either side of brushing your teeth.

Mobility Snacking Habit Stacking

At the start of the book, we nibbled on the idea of mobility snacking: little movement snacks sprinkled throughout the day to break up long periods of stillness and stagnation and practise some movement skills. I'm not going to go through the whole rigmarole again; a quick rehash is all we need for these crucial movement cookies.

249

If I ask you to add 10 squats into your day, no matter how good your intentions, you'll likely forget. You're human and we all have millions of things going on. However, your day is already laced with so many little things you do regularly – habits that are already embedded in who you are, just like brushing your teeth. While this is quite a ubiquitous example, there will also be habits specific to you and your life, all of which present a sensational opportunity to stack a new movement habit alongside them. This way, rather than just expecting you to remember, your already ingrained habit acts as the trigger for you to get down and move. This is known as 'habit stacking'.

My challenge for you: *list the things you do every day, without fail.*

Here are some of mine:

- Brush my teeth
- Make tea and coffee
- Feed my cat
- Put on my shoes
- Walk up and down the stairs
- Make lunch and dinner
- Take calls on Zoom
- Shower
- Get dressed
- Respond to emails
- Watch TV

That's a hell of a lot of opportunity to sneakily squeeze in some movement, alongside what I'm already doing anyway.

Here's what it could look like:

- Brush my teeth: 2 minutes of balance, 1 minute on each leg
- Make tea and coffee: 10 countertop push ups

- Feed my cat: 5 split squats
- Put my shoes on: old man test
- Walk up and down stairs: world's greatest stretch on the stairs
- Make lunch and dinner: squat every time I open the fridge
- Take calls on Zoom: sit on the floor or stand up for my calls
- Shower: shoulder dislocates with my towel
- Get dressed: hands behind the back floss with my T-shirt
- Respond to emails: hold the 90 90 or deep squat
- Watch TV: couch stretch and seated good mornings

I don't recommend doing all of these – that's a quick way to feel overwhelmed. I just want to highlight how many opportunities you have to move, right in front of your eyes, all ready to be exploited for your gain with minimal effort on your part.

To begin with I'd choose around 1–3 habits to stack and aim to nail them for a week. Once I felt comfortable with these, I'd then look at adding another, and another, until my day became riddled with wiggles.

It's likely when you embark on your mobility munching mission that you'll fly out the gates with wonderful intentions, but within half a day you'll have forgotten to do any squats, and you'll find yourself wondering what the point is. Fear not, my forgetful friend. We just have to pre-empt our forgetfulness and make it as hard to ignore as possible.

Post-It Notes

These small but mighty squares of fluorescent paper have an incredible power to remind us to do things we said we were going to do, especially when put in the right place. To help make these habitual moves even harder to ignore, scribble your mobility snack mission onto a Post-It note and place it right next to where you'll be when you should be busting out your move. If you're thinking 'I can ignore a Post-It note too', then write 10 of them, in bright pink, and include some positive encouragement too (or negative reinforcement if you're that way inclined). Make it so obvious that it's staring you in the face, and make a promise to yourself to commit to these snacks for two weeks. You won't have to cover your house in Post-It notes forever, but in the early days of your habit building, surrounding yourself with reminders and the odd bit of positive encouragement will work wonders for bringing these moves to the forefront of your mind.

Include Your Loved Ones

There aren't many things in the world we truly do on our own, even though it might feel like it. Most things we do day to day involve help from someone, somewhere down the line. Even just making a cup of tea uses electricity, a kettle, a tea bag, a mug and milk, all produced and supplied by others. We're connected little cookies who thrive in community, but when it comes to fitness it can often feel as though it needs to be a solo mission. But if you're trying to spark some good movement and health habits in your life, it's really helpful to lean on the people around you for support, accountability, or even to get involved with you.

If your immediate thought is that the people around you aren't going to support you, give them a try – they might surprise you. If not, then use their lack of support as fuel to find people who will. The world is full of people who want the best for you, even if they're not around you right now. Join a club, a community, connect on social media, and put yourself out there to find people who share the same mission as you. You might not find them straight away, but keep seeking because they're out there, I promise. A supportive community has consistently been shown to have a positive impact on exercise adherence.[1,2] It might be as simple as a pat on the back from a loved one, an exercise buddy, someone to walk with, or a class to join that helps keep your moving. Regardless of what it is, any opportunity you have to lean on others and share your movement journey and experience will make the world of difference.

Habits aren't set in stone; they're going to change and mould alongside your life. You don't have to be perfect all the time to make progress – far from it. Life has too many variables to expect your plan to go perfectly. Instead, embracing imperfect action, focusing on always doing something over 'all or nothing', and aiming for a version of consistency that suits your life will always win. Hopefully, these tips and tricks will give you a few ideas to help work some movement consistency into your life in a way that works for *you.*

Strut Your Stuff (Walking)

It ain't going to be news to any of you that walking is pretty bloody good for us; in fact, I'd go as far as to say it's the most underrated exercise of all time.

Our body is quite literally designed to waltz through the world on two feet. Everything from the position of our heads, the shape of our spines and hips, all the way down to our feet has been tailored to make us effective walkers. Walking is so central to our survival as humans that even our muscles are designed to help pump blood back to our heart as we walk and run.[3]

Of course, traversing around on two feet is a well-established beacon of physical and mental wellbeing support,[4] and something that anybody with a pair of legs can do. Plus, you're already doing it every day.

Not only will strutting your stuff keep the ticker ticking, the feet feeting, hips hipping, spine swaying and brain braining (these aren't official terms), the thing that makes walking amazing is how readily available it is. All you need to do is stand up and strut. And when it comes to mobility, motion is lotion. So, any form of movement that we can easily repeat, that's going to get the heart pumping, keep the joints lubed up and nutrients flowing to our muscles, is going to work wonders for building and maintaining our mobility. Walking is truly the lowest hanging fruit of the mobility world.

You've probably heard that you should aim to get 10,000 steps in every day. While I'm a huge fan and I would *love* you to smash that number daily, there's nothing 'magic' about the 10,000-step mark. You certainly don't need to hit 10k every day to benefit. I think it's better to see it as 'the more you walk, the more benefit you get'. If you've ever wondered how much you'll benefit, a recent meta-analysis including almost 227,000 people over an average of seven years identified that each 1,000-step increase in daily count was associated with a reduced risk of all-cause mortality by 15 per cent, while a 500-step daily increase was associated with a 7 per cent reduced risk of a cardiovascular event.[5] Meaning, as little as 5–10 minutes of extra walking a day can significantly reduce your risk of dying or having a heart attack. That's a saucy amount of health benefit for a minuscule amount of time if you ask me. Tracking steps is a sensational way of monitoring your overall activity levels, and striving for 10,000 steps is an amazing goal and one I encourage all of you to do your best to move towards, but remember that 4,000 is still a 100 per cent increase from 2,000, and has been shown to be enough to significantly reduce risk of all-cause mortality. So even if you're nowhere near hitting 10k, but you're improving on your baseline, you're doing a phenomenal job.

If you're a certified desk-dwelling diva, rooted to your desk eight hours a day, it might feel impossible to hit 10k steps some days, so try not to get too hung up on the numbers. When we measure movement solely by that metric, it can make the idea of a 200-step shuffle around your home or office seem insignificant – but that couldn't be further from the truth. Every time you stand up and shuffle, regardless of how far or how fast, you contribute to a more mobile body.

If you want to build a body that lasts, aim to improve your daily step count, regardless of where you start, and make sure you don't overlook the impact of regularly unfurling from your prawn posture and shuffling around, even if it's literally for a minute or two at a time. Do it as often as possible, ideally while still getting your work done. If your boss starts moaning at you for meandering a little too much, you can politely inform them that regular movement breaks have been shown to improve concentration and focus and will likely make you more productive.[6,7] Healthier and a more effective professional? Win win.

If you're looking to make a change, don't feel the need to rush to 10,000 steps overnight. Drastic changes in behaviour are often the most unmanageable in the long term, and if you haven't walked much for a while then your feet (and the rest of your body) will need a little time to adjust. Instead, aim to increase by 5–10 per cent each week, every couple of weeks or even each month, and try to spread your steps across the day as much as possible rather than doing them all in one big go.

Whatever you do, strut your stuff whenever you can, and every time you stomp your feet remember that you're contributing to a happy, healthy heart, head and home (body).

Butt, I'd Like You to Meet the Floor

When was the last time you sat on the floor? Back in those primary school days our bums were best pals with the floor, but for most of us in the Western world we've become estranged. I bet if you went to your mate's house and sat on the floor, they'd immediately offer you a chair, whereas in Asia or the Middle East, sitting on the floor is a lot more customary. I'd like to preface this by saying there's nothing wrong with chairs, but moving more throughout the day is about finding easy ways to sprinkle a little more mobility into our lives and there aren't many simpler ways than just sitting on the floor. So, while we think about the floor's potential to shape our ability to move, I'd like you to humour me and get that butt of yours on the floor. As in right now. If you're out in public at the moment, even better.

Chances are it won't be long before you get a little uncomfortable in whichever position you've popped yourself in, and before you know it, you'll have to shuffle into a different arrangement. Compare that to our comfy desk chairs and sofas, which most of us can perch on unperturbed for hours, and it soon becomes obvious why the floor is such a useful mobility tool for the lower body. It basically spurs regular movement, which as we know is the key to mobility. Sitting on the floor forces our ankles, knees and hips specifically into positions they don't otherwise find themselves in, and when it comes to floor dwelling, no one position is better than another. You have licence to shuffle around as much as you need from position to position.

Shift from your butt to the 90 90, then on to your knees. Or from your butt into a deep squat to lying on your side. Or roll your hips and butt around the floor while tapping away at your laptop, watching TV or eating dinner. This nearly constant state of movement while sitting on the floor is a habit that can reap some serious mobility rewards (I learned it from Dr Kelly Starrett @thereadystate, and it's one of the most wonderfully simple tricks in my personal mobility tool belt). Even 10 minutes here or there can have an incredibly positive effect on your lower body mobility.

Top tips for Desk-Dwelling Divas and Shift-Working Senors and Senoritas

Making mobility more of a focus when you spend the majority of your life rooted to your desk or stuck standing still for most of the day can be a sticky predicament, but there are plenty of ways to use this time to work on your movement ability. So, if you're a desk-dwelling diva, a home-working honey or a shift-working senor or senorita who's always on their feet, here are a few of my top mobility tips that you can wiggle into your day.

Get Comfy

My mate once said to me, 'Invest in your mattress and your shoes, because if you're not in one, you'll probably be in the other.' This doesn't mean you have to spend hundreds of pounds on a pair of trainers, but if you're on your feet all day it's worth exploring some comfy options and slapping them on your feet – and I'll extend this to your office chair, too! Explore what feels good for you. There's nothing worse than being uncomfortable for long periods of the day.

Change Places and Get Footloose

Hopefully by now you're conditioned like Pavlov's dogs and have already shimmied into a different position just from seeing the words 'CHANGE PLACES'. Remember, it's not that sitting is bad or that standing is good – it's doing nothing and being still for too long that's the issue. Regularly changing places is a great way of changing the demands on your body. Shuffle in your chair as much as possible and sit in all kinds of different positions throughout the day. Lean from side to side, and alternate the legs you cross and how you cross them. Lean back, sit upright, and prawn (I'm committed to making this a verb). These regular change ups will keep the stiffness at bay when you can't get away from your desk.

If you're standing, make sure you shuffle about and change position whenever you feel uncomfortable. You know those people that stand outside Buckingham Palace with the tall fluffy hats who just don't move all day? Don't be like them. You're not a statue, you're a human who needs to move, and standing still all day probably won't leave you feeling too fresh. This doesn't mean you have to run round in circles all day, but any opportunity you get to change your standing posture will likely keep the juices flowing and the muscles working in a variety of ways. You could lean on one leg, then the other, rest your foot or knee on a stool or a step, lean on a wall or a counter, or even sit down if you get a chance.

Different Workstations

Where possible, try to find different places in which to set up to work, whether it's at your desk, at a standing desk, sat on the floor with your laptop on a chair, or on a sofa. I set 30-minute timers to help me focus on getting my work done in chunks; every time they go off, I move to a different location in my house or change my desk from standing to sitting. (I'm lying by the way, I don't do this *every* time, but I try not to sit still for long.) This helps keep the cobwebs off and helps with focus too!

Stretch at Your Desk

There are plenty of chair-friendly stretches you can whip out to keep your body moving. You don't need a full fancy routine, just a handful of stretches you can cycle throughout the day. I always have a resistance band next to my desk to take my shoulders through some dislocates and to floss my hands behind my back.

Stood up all day? Touch your toes. Do a squat and hold it for a bit, maybe even a split squat if you're feeling really saucy. Need to pick something up? Do a single leg Romanian deadlift. Practise your balance. Take your shoulders for a spin and make some big circles with your neck. You might look a bit weird every now and again, but who cares – it'll help your body feel better!

Regular Movement Breaks

Sometimes you've just got to embrace the immortal words of Craig David, the godfather of garage, say, 'I'm walking away', and take a break from the desk. It doesn't have to be long, but it should ideally be regular. Stand up, have a shuffle, a shake, a wiggle, and just *move*. The same goes for my shift-working pals that may be in a stationary position for hours on end. You might not be able to sit down, but you can wiggle some extra movement variety into your day. Simple things like taking your neck, shoulders and hips through some big circles will work wonders. These small but regular movement breaks will go a long way to stave off the joint stagnation.

Work and Walk

I know lots of you won't be able to do this, but if you have regular meetings, why not take one while you walk rather than being sat in an office? If you're chairing the meeting, set the tone and lead by example. You'd be surprised how much more you get from your staff this way. Alternatively, if you have the luxury to invest in a walking pad, one of those mini treadmills for your home office, stick it under a standing desk and *voilà*. You'll be blown away how quickly the steps rack up. This has, without a doubt, been one of the greatest purchases I've made as a home working honey that's screwed to the laptop. It's the closest thing I can think of to a 'life hack' for getting steps in and something I one million per cent recommend!

Out of Office Hours

If you have no choice but to be wired to your desk or stationary on your feet all day, there isn't a lot you can do while you work, bar shuffling as much as possible, becoming a fidget, and taking the odd movement break when your schedule allows. I'm not going to tell you to quit your job just so you can move a little more during the day, that's a bit extreme (unless you hate your job, then I absolutely recommend finding one you hate less). If this is you, working hard at building movement routines outside of your working hours has to be a priority if you want your body to stay up to scratch. Walking to work, 10 minutes of morning movement, a few workouts a week . . . these dedicated movement sessions are going to be essential for giving your body the stimulus it needs to keep it ticking, but also taking the opportunity to move when it's put right in front of you. Next time you're on an escalator, walk up it rather than standing still, or better yet, take the stairs. If you need to go into town, walk rather than drive, or park a mile away and walk the rest. If you see a bench in a park, get your leg up and bust out the world's greatest stretch and maybe a split squat or two. The world is filled with opportunities to move, we just have to recognise them and seize them when they're there.

Injury Prevention

Injury prevention is an interesting term. To some degree, I believe that improving your mobility will help prevent injuries, or at least potentially reduce the risk or severity, depending on the activity. After all, increasing your flexibility and developing strength and coordination is likely to help you manoeuvre your way through any compromising positions you may find yourself in, whatever they may be (I'm not here to judge), by improving the resilience of your joint tissues. The issue with the term 'injury prevention' is that no matter how mobile you are, sometimes shit just happens. Even the most mobile of us can stub our toe, break a bone, or be hit by a car (touch wood that never happens). There are so many ways we can get injured, and unfortunately, picking up a minor or major niggle is an unavoidable part of life. It's important to know that you can be incredibly mobile and in pain and lack mobility while being pain free.

How Does Injury Happen?

The simplest way to look at the mechanics of injury is to understand that we all have a certain amount of 'load' or 'stress' that our body can tolerate. Let's call this our 'load capacity'. This applies across all of our body's tissues – the muscles, tendons, ligaments, bones, heart, and even our brain. When that load exceeds our body's tolerance, *bam*. You're going to get hurt.

Whether it's an acute injury like breaking a bone that happens suddenly, or a chronic injury that builds over time like tennis elbow, shin splints or plantar fasciitis, exceeding our body's capacity to tolerate stress leads to problems. It's pretty obvious why we want to avoid injury as much as possible – injuries suck, and the less time we spend injured, the more time we can spend honing our movement craft and going about our life. That being said, while it's good to avoid injury 'at all costs', it doesn't mean we have to become a hermit crab and avoid all activity out of fear.

Life is full of risks, and if you're human, you will probably get injured at some point. It really helps to understand and accept that it's totally normal to get injured, while remembering your body is a literal healing machine with an incredible ability to recover from seemingly catastrophic damage. Still, it's a pretty good idea for us to learn how to manage the amount of stress we put our bodies under, so we can help to mitigate this risk where possible. This is what we call 'load management'. It's impossible to give a perfect, one-size-fits-all guide to how to manage load, so instead I'm going to give you my 'load management 101' run down, and a template to help find your own personal Goldilocks Zone of bodily stress.

Load Management 101

In basic terms, load management is a balancing act between how much we train, known as our 'volume', how hard we train, known as our 'intensity', and our ability to recover. When we talk about 'stress', it's often seen as a bad thing, but like most things in life, the dose makes the poison. Too much stress is absolutely a bad thing and can lead to a shit storm of issues down the line, mentally and physically. But the 'right' amount of stress is needed to stimulate change and to help us grow. This amount is obviously going to be different for everyone based on several factors, including genetics and your training level, but, as a simple rule, just remember that when it comes to training, more doesn't always equal better. There's a fine line between building up your load capacity and overstressing yourself unnecessarily, and that is something we will explore below.

To find the right balance, we're looking at managing three main factors:

1. How often and how much movement you're doing (volume)
2. How hard you're exercising (intensity)
3. Your tolerance (how well you recover and your overall capacity for stress)

Because there's not a one-size-fits-all chart or formula, nor a perfect answer for how much, how hard and when to stop, here are two incredibly useful templates you can use to develop a better understanding of how you can personally balance the trio above.

The 8/10 'Rule' of Thumb

I put 'rule' in inverted commas because it's not really a rule at all, it's more of a guideline to help you work out roughly what should be enough and what might be too much when it comes to exercise intensity. Contrary to the popular 'no pain, no gain' or 'stay hard' mantras, I don't think many of us ever really need to push ourselves to 100 per cent effort in order to benefit from movement and exercise. I like to err on the side of caution when it comes to deciding how hard we should go, and suggest for most of us it's better to do a little too little than a little too much, especially in the beginning.

With training, it is far easier to add more over time than it is to take away, once you cross the 'too much' threshold. It's also a lot less daunting mentally. My general 'rule' of thumb is that nothing needs to be any harder than an 8/10 on our intensity scale (go to page 40 for a reminder of exactly what this looks like). This obviously doesn't mean that you'll immediately break if you push yourself beyond that level – in fact it's good to push every now and again to see what you're capable of. But as a blanket recommendation, I believe that 8/10 is a sweet spot to aim for. An 80 per cent intensity is still considered a vigorous effort, and it's a level that will be challenging enough to get you going and growing, but it's a reminder that not every exercise session has to be a 100 per cent 'I think I'm going to explode and die' kind of effort. If you're approaching training like that, it'll likely be a little too intense on the ol' recovery demands.

8/10 = Working hard but saving a little juice in the tank.

Now we have a simple template to guide us on how hard, here's another saucy blueprint for helping work out when to pull your socks up and get on with it and when you should chill your beans.

How Much Juice is in My Battery?

The body is a little like a battery. There are things we do that will drain us, and things that will help us recharge, and we want to make sure we have a good balance of both. If we constantly do things that drain our battery without ever taking time to top it up and recover, our stress tolerance will drop dramatically and leave us more susceptible to injury. Exercise itself has both the ability to charge our battery but also to deplete it, and I think which way that goes depends on when and how hard we choose to move. I've found an incredibly useful way to mediate this is to simply ask myself: 'What per cent is my battery at right now?'

This is a rough guide to how I'd recommend you approach exercise based on your answer.

Low Battery: 1–30%

(If you're wondering why it doesn't go down to 0 per cent, it's because 0 = dead.) If you're anywhere in this zone, you're going to feel *fatigued.* When it comes to improving any aspect of fitness, we need stress and rest in order to stimulate growth, and this is your sign to *rest.* Pushing yourself at this moment will likely cause an unnecessary increase in stress. If you want to move, which can help re-energise you, keep it super light intensity, like going for a stroll, a gentle stretch or very light workout. Movement will still be good for you, but the focus here should be to rest. Prioritise a good night's sleep, nutritious food and minimise other stresses in your life where possible. In this case I'd recommend you recharge your battery and come back another day.

Medium Battery: 30–70%

You're a bit tired, you don't feel your freshest, but you're not exhausted. Maybe you didn't have a great night's sleep, maybe you're a little stressed with work, but overall you're functioning fine. This is where the 'to move or not to move' question really matters, and my default answer is yes you should (shock) but with a minor caveat.

I'm sure you've heard people say they never regret a workout, and they always feel better afterwards. I *almost* always feel better after moving. But there will be the odd time when I've felt tired at the beginning of a workout and even worse by the end. To help you decide which way to go, here's what I'd recommend . . .

Start. Rip the plaster off and get started, just take it steady. If the battery feels a bit low, movement should be slow. If after 10 minutes you feel even lower on juice, go home. There is zero point in forcing it, and you should focus on recharging those batteries and come back tomorrow. It's important to give yourself permission to bugger off home and get some rest without feeling guilty for sacking off your workout. Be proud of yourself for starting, and even prouder for listening to your body. If after 10 minutes you feel better, then well done for getting started – it was totally worth it, wasn't it? Just remember to keep the intensity in check. You don't need to wrap yourself in cotton wool, but there's no need to go beyond 8/10 today. In fact, don't be afraid to keep even more in the tank and go for 6–7/10 if you feel you need to. You'll still get loads of benefit, without draining the battery any further.

High Battery: 70%+

You're flying, baby! You feel GOOOOOD. Okay, maybe not perfect, but your energy levels are up there. You slept well, ate well and you're feeling fine. Today's the day to push. Though just to be clear, you don't *have* to push yourself; you can still make improvements on your 8/10 trajectory. But if you fancy seeing what you're capable of and gunning towards a 9/10, maybe even 10/10, today's the day to try and set that PB (personal best, not peanut butter).

Similar to the intensity scale, this isn't about being as accurate as possible. It's about taking a moment to check in, see how you're feeling, listening to yourself, and adjusting accordingly.

Rather than treating yourself like a movement machine that always needs to be in 'Go' mode, it's about connecting with your very own scale. This system isn't perfect, but it's a lovely starting point from which to develop a more in-tune relationship with your body, setting yourself up for long-term bodily success and reducing the risk of avoidable injury. Over time, you'll start to note the signs when your battery is running low, medium or high.

When my battery is running low, I start to feel physically run down. I get a headache, a slightly blocked nose, claggy throat, the odd spot appears, and I feel *tired*. When this starts coming on, I take it as my sign to slow down, rest and recover. The opposite is true for when my battery is high. I feel bouncy, energetic, happy and enthusiastic, and I take these as signs to go like a little Duracell bunny. Pay attention to your own personal signs, because your body is amazing at telling you what it needs. Of course, it helps if we're listening, and even more if we're actively asking the question.

This is a great time to take a moment and reflect on your personal signs of a low life battery – those that you're already aware of, and those that maybe you've missed in the past.

While we can never truly 'prevent' injury (life happens), we absolutely can build our body's capacity to tolerate load, and we do this through training. Regularly exposing our body to loads that challenge us, but that we can tolerate, is how we stimulate our body to adapt over time. But that doesn't mean that more is always better for you every day of the week.

Try to see yourself as the puppet master of your stress. While there will *always* be external forces acting upon you that are out of your control, your job is to pull the necessary strings and adjust accordingly, based on what you need there and then. Perhaps that's more rest and recovery, or maybe it's a little more of a push.

DOMS

In case you're not familiar with DOMS, this cute little acronym stands for 'delayed onset muscle soreness', which usually rears its head 24–72 hours after exercise, and is best known for making life more difficult than it needs to be – especially when it comes to walking up and down stairs and sitting on the toilet. While this isn't an 'injury' per se, it can definitely feel like one. Fortunately, DOMS isn't always a default, or totally debilitating, response to exercise, with the effects ranging from 'slightly stiff' to 'oh God, what is wrong with my body?!' But why does DOMS happen in the first place?

DOMS is totally normal and you won't die from it, even though it might feel that way at the time. This spicy sensation can be a great feedback system, so here's everything you need to know about it.

There are a few theorised mechanisms of why our muscles scream at us post-exercise, but without getting too deep into the research of how it happens, soreness will normally appear after:

a. You do an exercise you haven't done before, or in a while

b. You do more than normal (an increase in volume or intensity)

The magnitude to which you feel DOMS will mainly be influenced by B, the intensity.

A certain level of soreness is to be expected post-exercise, especially in the beginning as your body works out what the hell you're doing to it and what it needs to do in response. The good news is that over time, as you repeat the same exercises again and again, your body gets used to the movements and the intensity of the soreness subsides.

I won't lie, I quite like the soreness. It's almost a 'hey, muscles, I know you've been working' kind of feeling that I find quite satisfying, but there's a tipping point at which this mild and weirdly satisfying soreness becomes debilitating and almost unbearable – usually when it starts to get in the way of simple things like putting your socks on or straightening your arms. This is usually a sign that you've done a little too much, a little too soon. Thankfully your body is an amazing healing machine and after a few days it'll return to normal, so there's no need to panic or give up completely, as the DOMS won't be as bad the next time you do the same workout.

To help mitigate the DOMS doom, when starting an exercise regime I encourage you to have a two-week 'acclamation phase'. Simply put, for the first two weeks of any new programme or activity – go easy. I'd recommend no more than a 5–6/10 on your intensity scale for the first week, 6–7/10 on the second week, and then up to your 8/10 sweet spot on the third week. This won't get rid of the soreness completely – you should still know your muscles have been worked – but it should reduce the likelihood of them feeling like they've been beaten to a pulp by giving your body a chance to acclimatise to the new exercise stimulus. Within a month or two of repeating the same exercises, you'll likely find your body stops getting sore from these movements altogether, or at least mostly – hooray!

All of us will overreach and dip our toe a bit too aggressively into the exercise waters at some point, then be smacked in the face (or arms or legs) by DOMS. This is especially the case if you set your sights on fitness feats such as running marathons, or anything that pushes your physical ability to the max, though it can also come from seemingly less intense pursuits that are a drastic deviation from our norm, such as a big day of walking or moving house. In these cases, there's little you can do to mitigate the DOMS, bar being patient and waiting for your body to do its thing, but there are a couple of things you can do to aid your recovery in the meantime.

If you possibly can, keep moving, even though it might not be 100 per cent comfortable. You'll probably find the soreness is at its worst when you stop and then start again, but once you're moving, you'll likely find the sore feeling isn't as intense. Gentle, continual movement will deliver the bloody, nutrient-filled goodness to the tender muscles, helping them recover quicker, and is known as 'active recovery'. So, if you're feeling beaten up, it's a good idea to get moving – it'll help!

In addition, focus on getting a good night's sleep, eating plenty of nutritious food, or if you're feeling really saucy you can get a little heat exposure in a sauna or a hot bath, which you may also find helpful.

Soreness isn't an indicator of an effective workout, but it is a sign that you're working. You should expect some soreness, but if you're continually feeling battered and bruised, it's worth looking at scaling back your intensity in the short term and prioritising your recovery a little bit better.

If you're unsure whether you should train while sore, firstly check in with your battery levels and see how you're feeling. But my general guidance is: if you're feeling absolutely banged up and it feels impossible, take the day off and go for a walk or have a gentle stretch instead and come back guns blazing tomorrow. If you're just a bit sore, then crack on! Training will likely help, so get to it.

Warming Up

We've all heard that we should warm up before we exercise to prevent injury, but is it true? And if so, what's the best way to warm up?

There's a bunch of research that shows warm ups improve performance,[1] but interestingly there's mixed evidence when exploring the link between warm ups and reduced risk of injury. Surprising, aye? Now this doesn't mean that warm ups don't reduce the risk, it just means we're not sure if they do or not. In fact, there are a few studies that do indicate a reduced risk.[2,3] Even though the research is a little inconclusive, it certainly doesn't hurt to warm up. Either way, it's guaranteed to help you perform better, so what's not to love?

What Should a Warm Up Look Like?

If you're looking to maximise performance, I'd recommend dividing a warm up into three parts to get the best outcome:

1. A pulse-raising activity to get your core temperature up. A good guide is exercising until you are lightly sweating. This will look different for everybody, but a simple suggestion could be 5–10 minutes of brisk walking.
2. Dynamic stretches. Dynamic just means moving, so any movements that are going to get the muscles and joints you're about to use lubed up will be fine. This could literally be as simple as arm and leg swings, and I'd recommend spending a few minutes giving your limbs a good old go around until they feel nice and warm.
3. Perform the activity you're about to do but at a lower intensity. Going for a run? Start with a brisk walk or jog. About to do some heavy squats? Do some light squats. About to do some push ups? Start with some incline push ups (hopefully you get the point).

This is what I'd consider an 'optimal warm up', as it's likely to help you get the best results out of your activity. In reality, I know you won't always have time to bust out a full warm up, and the last thing I want is for this to become a barrier or a reason not to do your workout.

If you're short on time and just want to get cracking, there's no need to spend 20 minutes warming up, just focus on performing the activity you're about to do, but at a lower intensity for a couple of rounds (number 3 on the list above) with a small break in between. Ideally, you will then gradually increase the intensity with each round until you're at your working effort (your 8/10). This will get your core temperature up and prepare your body for exercise, but in as little time as possible. If you want to milk as much mobility juice out of this mini warm up as you can, I'd recommend also introducing some static or dynamic stretches during your breaks on any of your restricted areas, e.g. a 90 90 in between your squats to help open up your hips. Just aim to keep any static stretches to 30 seconds (or less); that way the stretches won't negatively impact your strength.[4]

To make it nice and easy for you, the programmes I've recommended have been designed with the exercises ordered in a way that will warm you up as you go, so there's no need to do extra beforehand – just dive right in and follow the order. And there is no need to warm up before mobility snacks – the whole point is that these snacks are to be nibbled on throughout the day at a lower intensity to 'grease the grooves', rather than at max effort!

Injury, Recovery and Working Around Pain

Being injured is miserable, but if that's you right now, not all hope is lost. There will still be things you can do to both maintain and improve your mobility, and also speed up your recovery, depending on the injury; and with a little shift in perspective this can be a beautiful opportunity to learn more about your body.

This isn't intended to be medical advice. As always, speak with your physician or medical professional before engaging in any of these practices. Below I am going to offer you some tips on where to start if you're coming up against injuries based on my experiences as a personal trainer that's also navigated his fair share of injuries, and the top lines in the current research.

If you're dealing with a soft tissue injury (muscle, ligament, tendon, etc.), you've likely been recommended RICE at some point. I'm not talking about those delicious white grains that accompany your favourite curry or sushi, I'm talking about the acronym: Rest, Ice, Compression, Elevation.

Whether for a sprained ankle or a knackered knee, most of us have been told to slap some ice on it and rest as soon as possible. But it turns out the RICE godfather himself, Dr Gabe Mirkin, actually recanted this recommendation in 2015. After almost 40 years, it now turns out that icing and complete rest may actually *delay* healing by preventing inflammation, an essential part of the healing process.[1] So not only does RICE not work, it might even make your injury last for longer.

Fear not, my newly mobile friends, because I am here to help you bid *adieu* to RICE and hello to PEACE and LOVE (sounds nicer, doesn't it?).[2] This cuddly new acronym encourages a more movement-centric approach to recovery. Sounds good, right?

For the first few days of injury (days 1–3) we want some PEACE:

P = Protect. Avoid activities and movements that increase pain for a couple of days after injury. This doesn't mean stop all movement completely. We want to get the injured area moving as soon as possible, if only gently, a tiny amount, without causing extra pain.

E = Elevate. Lift your injured limb higher than your heart.

A = Avoid anything anti-inflammatory. Inflammation helps the healing process, so there's no need to stock up on Ibuprofen!

C = Compress. Wrap it up.

E = Educate. Empower an active recovery approach to injury, just like we're doing right now.

Once those first few days have passed, we need a little LOVE:

L = Load. It's time to get the tissues working again by introducing some low-intensity exercise to the injured area. In other words, get it moving with some minor manageable movement. This keeps the blood flowing, bringing the nutrients needed for recovery to the area. Be guided by your pain; it's likely to hurt a little, but it should be tolerable. Imagine a doctor asked you how bad your pain was out of 10 – we want to keep roughly within 3/10 on this pain scale. If >3/10, scale back the intensity and if it's unbearable, see a doctor!

O = Optimism. Optimistic people generally have better outcomes. Focus on the positives. You're alive – hooray!

V = Vascularisation. A fancy way of saying, get the cardio in. This will help keep you fit, aiding your recovery and return to activity.

E = Exercise. Exercise will help build strength in the damaged tissue, while restoring mobility and coordination. In an ideal world, this would be guided by a medical professional such as a physio or physical therapist.

In short, after a few days of rest, it's good to get the injured tissue working again. Starting with light, minor weight-bearing activities that generate minimal pain to the area, what you want to do is find other ways to keep the blood moving and the heart delivering goodness to the injured area.

While you're recovering and introducing a little PEACE and LOVE to the damaged area, focus on working other body parts. If it's an ankle injury, work on your hips, spine and shoulders. If it's a leg injury, work the other leg. In the latter case, there's even some research that suggests that working the non-injured limb may help maintain muscle mass, through something known as 'cross education', and may also maintain a stronger brain–body connection with the injured limb. So if you find your right arm in a cast, training your left arm probably won't grow your right arm, but it will likely help the injured limb return to activity sooner (yay).[3]

The wonderful news is that your body is a literal healing machine, and most minor muscular skeletal injuries will fix themselves over time, without you having to do anything drastic, or really anything at all. But sometimes pain pops up without an obvious injury and this can be really bloody annoying, especially when it gets in the way of doing things you love to do, so here are some of my top tips for working around a painful movement, to help keep you moving and doing what you love.

Working Around a Painful Movement

Pain is a complex topic. So complex that it would need its own book – multiple, in fact – to cover it from every angle. Books that I'm definitely not qualified or educated enough to write, and which probably wouldn't even scratch the surface of the complexity. But the last thing I want is you a) hurting yourself unnecessarily, or b) avoiding movement completely out of fear. So, if you've found any of these movement challenges (or any exercise) painful, here's an approach to help you navigate the pain, and hopefully helping you to mitigate it without stopping you moving or doing the exercise entirely.

I've often wondered if everyone sees the same blue that I see. The chances are, across the eight billion of us on the planet, that the answer will most likely be 'no'. I believe the same applies for how we experience pain. Pain is a spicy and unpleasant sensation (not that you need reminding), but bloody important, and one that is undoubtedly experienced with subtle differences from person to person. This makes creating a 'standardised model' for pain a little tricky.

Pain, of course, serves an evolutionary function. If you've ever grabbed something hot from the oven without an oven glove or tea towel, you'll be familiar with the searing pain that radiates through your newly fingerprint-less fingers. That pain singes more than your skin, stimulating your brain too, and acting as a stark reminder not to touch very hot things going forwards, because that shit hurts. We accumulate these potently painful reminders through individual experience (aka the hard way), and through thousands of years of evolutionary trial and error, which echoes through our human culture – which is rather useful in encouraging us not to be numpties.

This is why it can be incredibly difficult to return to an activity we once injured ourselves doing; we are hardwired to develop fear. The problem with our good pal pain is that it's not always the most reliable indicator of how much damage we've done. If you've ever rubbed antiseptic into a wound, you'll know how horrendously unpleasant and painful an experience it is, yet it doesn't cause any extra damage. Despite the pain, you're actually helping by cleaning the wound and protecting against infection. For this reason alone, we can't rely *solely* on pain as an accurate indicator of how much damage something is doing, or when something is 'bad'. Our objective is therefore not to avoid pain completely, but to develop a better relationship with it and better understand where this fine line lies.

How Much is Too Much?

The sort of painful feelings we want to avoid throughout these movement challenges (and life) are any sharp, stabbing sensations. Generally, anything that makes us go 'ouch' and recoil is not something we want to push through. I've often found when coaching people that these painful sensations are quite apparent, and you'll often *know* when you feel them. To help make it a little clearer, if I asked you to rate your pain out of 10, a good ballpark to aim for is 'no more than 3/10 on the pain scale'; anything over that and you're probably pushing too far, unnecessarily.

If you're new to the world of exercise, you haven't moved much in a while, or you're overcoming injury, you may find that you're a little more sensitive to pain than usual. Paired with our individual differences in how we experience pain, this may mean you meet your 3/10 a lot sooner than somebody who's been moving a lot more regularly, or somebody with a greater tolerance to pain. The important thing is to try stay within this 1–3/10 range, no matter how small those movements may seem at the beginning.

Remember, it's good to keep moving in any capacity. And over time, the more you explore your body's capabilities, not only will your understanding of where your 3/10 is become clearer, you may also find your body becomes less sensitive and you are able to tolerate a lot more at 3/10 than you once were. Don't be surprised if you have no idea where your 3/10 currently lies – nobody does to begin with. Like any language, learning takes time.

Reminder:
Moderate Pain Doesn't Always = Damage

If you dip your toe into movement and find yourself face to face with a little more pain than normal, I want you to feel as prepared as possible to manoeuvre yourself around it, rather than giving up altogether. I'm a firm believer that totally avoiding painful movement only leads to more issues down the line, as when we find ourselves dodging those movements it will lead to weaker joints and muscles in the long run, and a bigger hill to climb. Instead, we want to develop as many tools as possible to help us work around pain, so here's my five-step process to help you do this. You can use this process for any of the movement challenges that you've struggled with, to help adapt each one for your own needs. But you can also use it for almost *any* exercise you do out in the world. So when you tip over the 3/10 pain edge, you can try the steps below.

Step 1 – Slow Down

One issue when we're learning an exercise is that we often find ourselves focusing on the number of reps more than the quality of the movement and end up bouncing up and down like a yoyo, trying to rush through each rep. This isn't automatically 'bad', in fact explosive movements such as our pogos (page 130) are incredibly important for developing and maintaining spring-like qualities in our muscles and connective tissues, especially for sports that require power. But when it comes to mastering a movement that feels a little painful, and developing strong, healthy joints and muscles, it's a good idea to slow down in the beginning, especially on the way down. This 'bouncing' means we don't spend much time engaging the muscles and joints across the whole range of motion. Instead, we bounce from Point A to Point B with little control and purpose and miss out on a huge amount of benefit to our joints and muscles.

If you want to really develop strength across a movement, it helps to make sure the movement is controlled. Think about it like a lift (or elevator if you're American). If you were moving from the second floor to the first floor, you'd want it to be steady and controlled. If your lift flung you up and down carelessly, you wouldn't hesitate to take the stairs next time. It's the same for irritable joints. If you want to squeeze the most juice out of any movement, it will pay dividends to slow the movement down, especially on the way down, as you resist gravity. This is known as the *eccentric* part of the movement, in case you missed that part earlier. I'm not saying you need to start moving super slow, like you're David Hasselhoff or Pamela Anderson running down the beach in *Baywatch*. A 3–4-second descent will do the trick and hopefully make the movement hurt less.

Step 2 – Reduce the Load (Intensity) or Use Assistance

One of the greatest tips I can give for working around a painful movement is to reduce the intensity. This is all about reducing the stress on your tender bits and the easiest way of doing this is to lift less weight. Pick up a lighter weight or transition back to bodyweight until you're able to do at least 10–20 reps of any movement without pain. You can then look to make the exercise more challenging by picking up the smallest available weight increment and giving it another go.

If you're not using additional weight and are struggling to get into these movements with your bodyweight alone, we need to think a little more creatively by finding ways to add assistance. The easiest method of doing this is to find something to hold on to or something that can give you support. This may include using a suspension trainer, a type of equipment you can attach to a door frame or bar to provide assistance, or resistance bands. Or if you want to save your cash, in many cases you can simply find something like a chair, a door frame, or even another person to provide a little stability, and a surface to push or pull yourself up with.

As you gain confidence with the movement, over time you can start to rely less on the assistance of your chosen object and more on just using your target muscles to complete the movement.

If you get pain when walking or running, adding assistance isn't really an option, but reducing the load certainly is. You may find that when you walk or run that you're fine for the first mile, but by the time you get to the second mile your knee really starts to hurt. Instead of avoiding walking or running altogether, you can reduce the load by splitting the distance in half over two sessions and walking or running one mile at a time, rather than all in one. Every week look to increase your mileage, maybe by 5–10 per cent maximum, or as long as you can without pain. You'll likely find that by reducing the load but increasing the frequency, your body will have time to adjust, hopefully with less pain.

Step 3 – Reduce the Range of Motion

There are so many benefits to training your movements across their full range of motion, and hopefully I've encouraged you to do so throughout this book. But there's no need to rush. The tortoise wins the race, and you're a sexy tortoise. If it hurts when you go down low, or stretch far into a movement, there's a chance you may be going too far too soon. Next time you set up for an exercise, move slowly (Step 1) and pay attention to how far into the movement you get before it hurts and passes that 3/10 pain mark. Once you know where the tender bit is, stop *just before there*, pause for a couple of seconds, and then push yourself up. This approach is about developing confidence, control and coord-ination within ranges of motion we already possess, before looking at extending beyond and is incredibly underrated when it comes to improving our mobility. This is when filming yourself is helpful. Instead of pushing ourselves into pain, we want to focus on building strength in our pain-free range of motion. The stronger we get in this pain-free range, the easier it becomes to increase our range of motion over time.

For some exercises, you can also use physical objects to give feedback for how far you should go, for example by placing a chair under your bum when you squat. When you feel the object, you know you've gone far enough.

Step 4 – Tweak Your Technique

Technique is important for optimising performance. If you want to run as fast, jump as high or lift as much weight as possible, your technique absolutely matters. However, other than attaining peak performance, I don't think technique is as important as people make it out to be, assuming it's not putting you at immediate risk and that it doesn't hurt. If it does put you at risk or hurts, then you absolutely should look to change your technique, and if you've tried slowing the movement down, reducing the range of motion and using assistance but it still feels off, you need to play around with your body positioning. This is where filming yourself and getting external feedback can be incredibly helpful, rather than trying to identify the issue yourself. That being said, simple changes such as hand or foot position, or the way you move your hips, can make a world of difference in how a movement feels for you. Play around with what feels good, even if it doesn't look conventional. For years I tried to keep my back perfectly straight when doing a deadlift and it hurt every time. The moment I allowed myself to play with what felt comfortable for *me* and ignored the one-size-fits-all movement approach, I found a position that allowed me to lift pain free.

Step 5 – Try a Different Exercise or Activity

If you've tried the steps above and no matter how you adapt the move, it just hurts, try something else! Despite this book being filled with some of my favourite exercises to help build your movement ability, no one move is so important that you *must* do it. There are countless variations of different movements to try that work similar movement patterns, similar muscles, and with similar benefits that can be adapted to you and your needs. For each challenge I've listed easier variations of the exercises you can attempt to see if they feel better for you. The important thing is that you're exercising and finding what works, rather than avoiding something completely because it hurts. Also, just because one thing hurts, doesn't mean they all will. If that movement is important to you, instead of totally steering clear of it, you can adapt it and make it easier by finding a variation that you can do without pain, while simultaneously discovering a way to build up strength through Steps 1–3. Alternatively, if you just want to exercise but don't mind what you do, you can try an entirely different type of activity. There are infinite forms of exercise out there that you may love, that doesn't aggravate your tender bits, giving your body time to recover and come back to the original activity another day should you wish. By doing this, it means the body keeps working and, as we know, if we don't use it, we lose it. Whatever you do, don't stop moving.

Setbacks and Flare-ups

While we don't want to avoid pain completely, if you do find that working through an exercise or a workout causes a flare-up the next day and you find yourself in more pain than usual, that's a sign you've exceeded your body's tolerance. Most of the time these flare-ups will calm down by themselves with a bit of rest, but it's important to pay attention to what you were doing, how much and how hard you were working, in order to identify your current tolerance, so that when you come back to training, you can start with a smaller dose and build up from there. Reductions in pain may take time, or may calm down in a day or two, but if you're able to find a movement that you can perform within that 3/10 pain range and the next day your pain isn't any worse, that's a win as you've just got stronger without your pain increasing and you're on the right track.

If pain does persist and you're concerned, please do speak to a medical professional to rule out any major damage. As I made clear in the beginning, none of the information in this book is there as a substitute for medical advice, and the reality is that some of you may need further help to identify why you're dealing with discomfort, and to help you create a plan to overcome and work around it.

The Cup Analogy: Understanding Pain Better

An analogy I learned from Greg Lehman, which I've found incredibly helpful, compares pain to an overflowing cup.[4] The cup represents our ability to tolerate life's stresses; when the stressors build up beyond the size of your cup, that's likely when you'll experience pain. There are a lot of things that contribute to an overflowing cup, beyond the more apparent physical bits and bobs that you're made up of, like muscles, tendons, ligaments, discs etc. It could be physical stress, worry, poor sleep, nutrition, fear, loneliness, social isolation, or any other of your individual life loads. All of these things, and more, can contribute to the fullness of your cup, but we all have a tipping point where it gets a little too full. And when it does, it's probably going to hurt. So, when you're in pain, no matter how much you manipulate an exercise, it still hurts. It's important to remember that you're more than just a bag of meat and bones, you're a human being with lots of moving pieces in your lives. But there are two things you can focus on doing to help manage your pain.

1. Reduce the stressors in your life (what goes in the cup).
2. Build a bigger cup.

Only you will know what fills your cup. Asking yourself if there is something specific that needs to be addressed, identifying it (or them), and doing your best to minimise how much or how many of them you allow in your cup is a great start. But it also helps to look at building a comically sized mug, and anything you can do to improve your health and happiness will go a long way towards doing this.

So is there anything you can do to improve your health and your happiness? Hopefully you've found some in this book already, but if you are dealing with consistent pain and are unsure where to turn, I hope this encourages you to look at the big picture and ask yourself how you can build one big ol' cup and monitor what goes in there.

The Big Picture

When it comes to building a body that lasts, wiggling more movement into your life is an essential piece of the puzzle, but it's not the only piece. To become a truly mobile munchkin, now and for the long haul, you also need to throw your overall health and wellbeing into the equation and remember that you're not just a movement machine. You're a human being and more likely to thrive when your whole ecosystem is in good nick, and that's what these deliciously fruity additions are all about; simple ways of improving your overall health and wellbeing. In other words, how to build a bigger cup.

Catch Your Zs

I probably don't need to harp on about 'why sleep is important'. Our brain wouldn't shut down and temporarily paralyse us every night unless it really had to, and if you've ever found yourself a little sleep-deprived, I'm sure you'll appreciate how missing out on a deep rest can make the world of difference to how we function throughout the day. I'm a little demon when I haven't had my sleep.

Sleep is an essential component of health and recovery,[1] which makes it a fundamental pillar in our ability to move and heal. If we're chronically sleep-deprived, our ability to maintain our physical and mental capacity is going to go down the drain. I don't want to be too preachy when I waffle about the importance of sleep. I'm sure there's nothing more some of you would love than a good night's sleep, but due to working night shifts or taking care of kids or whatever it is that keeps you from your shuteye, it doesn't always come easy. Nor do I want to suggest that if you can't prioritise your slumber for whatever reason, that you'll suddenly break.

That being said, if you want to do as much as you can to support your health endeavours, prioritising sleep wherever possible will have a monumental impact on your ability to recover and function as a human being, as well as your motivation. Getting a workout in can feel like a grind at the best of times, but it can be especially tough when you're knackered.

Here are a few practical tips which may help you develop a more sustainable sleep pattern.

1. Set a bedtime and wake time, and try to stick to it (circadian rhythm, innit?).
2. Build a night-time routine to help you unwind.
3. Limit screen time an hour before bed.
4. Read a book.
5. Avoid caffeine from the afternoon onwards.
6. Do some exercise during the day.

Most of us are guilty of shunning an extra hour of sleep to squeeze more minute's doom scrolling on our phone or watching the seventh episode of a series in a row. While this probably won't touch the sides every now and again, if this is your default setting, you're not giving your body the time it needs to shut down, rest and recover. I ain't saying you need to obsess over every minute of sleep, but if I've described your bedtime protocol above and you want to take care of your body a little better, start here. These aren't the deepest of sleep tips, but it's often the simplest tips that are the most impactful, and these are great places to start.

Nutrition

I wasn't lying when I said these concepts weren't revolutionary. First sleeping. What's next, a healthy diet? Yep! That is *exactly* what I'm suggesting.

What you put in your mouth is the fuel you're supplying to your body. Similar to sleep, this fuel aids our ability to recover and provides us with energy to do the things we need to do. If we want our body to function well, it helps if we give it what it needs in order to get the best from it.

The world of nutrition can be an absolute minefield, with every other person shouting at you about what you should and shouldn't be eating. I have no interest in adding to the noise, but I would be doing you a disservice as a personal trainer on a well-being mission if I didn't at least give you some overarching guidance. Without going too deep into what's good and what's not, I'm going to keep this nice and simple.

Firstly, I don't believe any food in isolation is so bad that it will kill you (unless you're allergic to it, in which case, obviously don't eat it). Realistically, nobody develops heart disease or diabetes from a single doughnut or pizza. So when looking at the quality of someone's diet, it's important to look at the bigger picture. When it comes to the buzzword of the moment, 'ultra-processed' foods can be at least a small part of your life while still eating a 'healthy diet'. Not to be the Grim Reaper here, but you could eat perfectly 100 per cent of the time and you're still going to die. So there's no need to be a nutrition nun and abstain from any and all food-based enjoyment. Just try not to take the piss. Despite the deliciousness, a doughnut isn't the most nutrient-dense food compared to, say fruit, veg or whole, less processed foods. So while it's a good idea not to demonise individual foods, or whole food groups, it is absolutely a good idea to get as much goodness into your diet as you can, with a focus on nutritious plant-rich foods. It ain't rocket science, though I know that doesn't make it easy in practice because temptations are everywhere.

This is why I encourage all my clients to aim for '80 per cent whole foods, 20 per cent soul foods'. Aiming for 80 per cent – the majority of your diet – to be made up of minimally processed, nutritious whole foods is never going to be bad advice. And I'm not going to hold your hand here; I know you know what nutritious, healthy food is. However, 20 per cent of your diet should be made up of 'soul foods'. These are the foods that tickle your soul and make you murmur 'wawaweewa' under your breath as the taste tickles your lips. Food is more than fuel, it's imbedded in culture, socialising, memories, bonding – and it should be enjoyed. But you'd know you were pushing it if you ate nothing but chips and burgers. I'm sure your body won't mind me speaking on its behalf when I say it would appreciate some fruits and vegetables, even if you don't love the taste of them. For example, eating a Mediterranean diet, considered the model of healthy eating, has been associated with a lower decline in mobility and lower risk of mobility disability.[2]

This 80–20 diet split is not a *rule.* It's a guide to encourage you to eat more of the good stuff your body needs, while giving some flexibility to indulge in the things you really love. In reality, it's unlikely you'll actually stick to this split all the time. Sometimes life will get in the way and you'll have to grab food on the go, so maybe that 80–20 will shift to 60–40 for a week. Or maybe you're feeling a little run down and want to fuel yourself, so it shifts the other way to 90–10. Regardless of exactly where you aim with the nutritional split, if you want a healthy, happy bod that feels good, you're going to need to fuel it well. When it comes to low-hanging fruit, there isn't much lower than literal fruit.

In practice, this could simply mean:

- 1–2 extra pieces of fruit a day
- Vegetables with most meals
- Eating one or two biscuits, rather than the whole pack
- Drinking an extra glass of water a day

Literally Anything That Improves Your Health or Happiness

In case you're not catching my low-hanging fruity drift, what I'm trying to get across is that anything you can do that moves your health needle in a positive direction will likely improve how you move, now and in the future, simply by improving your overall wellbeing. And when I say anything, I mean *anything*. From hydration to minimising unnecessary stress to more sex – if you're focusing on improving your health, your mobility will benefit. You're more complex than just a bag of meat and bones that moves. You're an entire ecosystem with lots of moving pieces in the canvas of your health, and if you're ignoring the three fundamental pillars of walking, sleeping and eating entirely, you're likely trying to build a house on shaky foundations. This doesn't mean you need to become militant with your steps, sleeps and eats, but doing your best to identify small, simple, manageable improvements you can make to your overall health will go an incredibly long way to keeping you alive and kicking way down the line.

I know how overwhelming it can feel when someone throws a load of health suggestions at you in one go. If you're prone to feeling overwhelmed when it comes to shifting your health markers, let's make it a little easier by breaking them down one at a time.

What's one thing you can do this week to improve your health and wellbeing?

Here's a list of suggestions:

- Go for a walk every day.
- Set a step count goal that's 5–10 per cent higher than last week.
- Set a bedtime and stick to it.
- No screens an hour before bed, read a book instead.
- Eating an extra piece of fruit every day.
- Drink an extra glass of water every day.
- Do a workout from this book (or elsewhere).
- Spend some time with loved ones.
- Do something you enjoy.

Choose one of these or make one up for yourself – anything that's going to positively contribute to a healthier, happier you and focus on nailing that *one thing* this week. And then the following week, add another. You don't have to do everything at once; in fact, breaking it down means it's more likely to stick.

Hidden Benefits of Mobility Training

The aim of the mobility game is to wiggle your way through life, confident that your body is up to scratch and able to overcome the challenges and obstacles you meet along the way. There is an abundance of obvious benefits to a mobile body, but I've also discovered a few hidden gems that go above and beyond the bendiness, balance and general manoeuvrability.

While I care immensely about your physical movement abilities, I also have a soft spot for that brain of yours, and this exercise business has a way of positively nudging your mental wellbeing in the right direction, especially when life feels a little heavy (and even when it doesn't). But what I have learned is that movement doesn't just support your mental health, it also equips you with some mental faculties that can actually help overcome the inevitable challenges life throws your way.

It's really, *really* hard to 'switch off' from the world sometimes. Our attention has become currency, and everything is constantly trying to steal it from us, but that can come at a great cost to our mental wellbeing. It's no secret we're in a mental health crisis, and although I don't think that's because people aren't stretching enough, or that mobility training is the singular answer to much wider systemic issues that need to be addressed on a societal level, I do believe that tending to your physical needs gives you a doorway through which you can disconnect from the world. Focusing on your physical, bodily self instead of the noise all around you directs your attention internally for a moment.

Turning your focus towards yourself and your moving parts rather than the million other things going on in the outside world is a bit like releasing a pressure valve in the system.

As someone who has at times felt like I've had the weight of the world on my shoulders, I can say that it's far harder to feel overwhelmed by the past or the future when you're deep in a stretch. There is something about trying to focus on breathing through the physical discomfort that grounds you in the 'now'. Everyone is always banging on about being more present – well, I haven't found a better way to snap myself into the moment than really going for it in the 90 90, a split squat or the world's greatest stretch. It's hard to be on another planet when you're concentrating on the intense stretch in your groin. It's like accidental mindfulness. While I've always found mindfulness to be a bit of a contextless buzzword (my mind is full enough, thank you), I've found an inconceivable amount of benefit in occupying my mind with physical focus. It might sound like an avoidance tactic, but I've actually found my brain is a lot better at tackling problems when I give it space to breathe, rather than continually banging my head against the wall, cycling through the same thoughts again and again. Movement helps me stop the mental ruminations in their tracks.

I'll be the first to admit that stretching, strength training and exercise can be a tad boring at times, and I'll agree that when we're bored it's easier to fall back into the abyss of circular thoughts. This is why I've served you up so many different movement challenges and mobility snacks. If you're getting bored, just skip on to something new to keep it feeling fresh. What's more, if you can look past the boredom and dig a little deeper, even beyond the long-term physical benefits I've been rubbing in your face, you might find movement practices are more than just an avenue to build a robust body; they also build a more peaceful and resilient mind.

Essentially, this mobility game is one big problem-solving mission of understanding your body. A mission that only you can take on, and one that requires you to be a patient puppy and consistent cookie that keeps coming back, again and again and again, for as long as you can. Both patience and consistency – two invaluable life skills – are sharpened the deeper you dive down this movement rabbit hole.

Though much of this mobility malarkey is about paying into your movement pension, don't underestimate the immediate and long-term impact these wonderful wiggles have on that beautiful brain of yours. Next time you're feeling a little out of sorts, why not give your body a flex – you never know, it could totally change the trajectory of your day.

And in case you think I'm chatting out of my bum, the research seems pretty conclusive. This review of 15 studies including almost 200,000 people found that even small amounts of physical activity consistently led to significant mental health benefits and reduced association of depression.[1] A wiggle here and a wiggle there might not seem like much, but you'd be surprised to what degree it can help to release a bit of mental and physical pressure now and again.

Are you really going to make me ask? Okay, fine. If you could please BREATHE and CHANGE PLACES, that would be wonderful – thank you.

You're a Miracle

Well, well well . . . It looks like we've made it to the end (of this book). Hopefully this is far from *the end* and you and that body of yours have a long, beautiful life together, but before I say my goodbyes, I have some final thoughts to leave you with.

The world has changed a lot in the last hundred years, compared to the life our grandparents or great-grandparents knew. I'm obviously not speaking from personal experience, but I'm sure we can agree that in the grand scheme of our human she-nanigans, a century is a minuscule slice of time. To put into per-spective how ludicrously fast our world and technology has advanced over the last hundred years, let's talk about the Wright brothers. Those boys made history by completing the first ever successful flight in 1903, travelling 180 feet in just 12 seconds. Fast forward to 1969, and only 66 years later we'd gone from flying the length of two tennis courts to landing on the Moon, over 384,000 kilometres away – in a spaceship. It's been another 55 years since then, and even within that tiny window of time, we've seen what once would have been considered an inconceivable amount of change. The internet, email, smart phones, AI. We live in a totally different world.

Nostalgia aside, technology is evolving exponentially along-side the ever-changing world we live in, and it doesn't appear to be slowing down. Our world might have changed a lot in the last 100 years, but us? Not so much. Fundamentally, the anatomical bricks and mortar that make us human remain incredibly similar to the first *Homo sapiens* almost 300,000 years ago. There's no question our DNA is evolving too, but nowhere near as quickly. We simply haven't had the chance to catch up with the new demands of the world around us, and I believe it's about time somebody was honest in saying that *you* are not the problem.

I'm not convinced we need to start living like our hunter-gatherer ancestors, walking around barefoot 24/7 or eating a paleo diet. I'm a fan of supermarkets and shoes, and life's too short not to enjoy the odd doughnut. However, 100 – or even 50 – years ago, there would have been a very strong likelihood that you and I would have walked to work or to buy our food, and generally been on our feet more, partly because it would have been less usual for us to have owned a car. Now I wake up, I move from my bedroom to my living room, I open my laptop and jump on a Zoom call. Even though I'm a personal trainer, some days it gets to 6pm and I've walked less than a thousand steps between my sofa and my fridge.

That isn't to say that people in the past wouldn't have experienced issues with mobility, pain or injury – they absolutely did. It's more that movement was so ingrained and embedded in our lives. Whereas today, it just isn't. That being said, it's not your fault, nor mine, that most of us spend eight hours, five days a week, curled up at our desk like a prawn just to afford the roof over our heads and the bills that follow. We are all trying to do our best. While these wild changes to the world ain't our fault, I need you to know that although you're not the problem, you have the power to be the solution. If you decide to work on your mobility in the ways outlined in this book, you can help tackle the sedentary nature of the times we live in and build a body that lasts.

It may surprise you to know that, to all intents and purposes, I wasn't supposed to be here. Back in 1993, after the birth of my brother and sister, my parents decided they'd had enough little tiddlywinks (children) and concluded it was best to tie the knot – of the vasectomy variety. I never thought I'd write about my dad's testicles in a book, yet here we are. As you may already have concluded, the events that followed didn't unfold exactly as my parents had expected. To both my mother and father's shock, the vasectomy didn't work. I promise I do have a point here, and it is very simply the fact that I didn't choose to be here, and I can safely presume you didn't either. This just . . . happened. We're all innocent by-products of the romantic (or not so romantic) fumblings of our parents, their parents, their parents, and years and years of successful shagging throughout the millions of years of human existence.

I don't want to drag you too deep down a philosophical rabbit hole and spark an existential crisis, as I know you probably just bought this book to learn how to make your body feel better. But before I leave you to spread your mobility wings, I want you to appreciate something astounding. You, me and literally everyone else in the world, are the result of a ludicrously incomprehensible unbroken chain of events across 13.8 billion years of our universe's history. The chances of us being here, as a human being, on a rock flying through space at 1,600 kilometres per hour, around a ball of fire almost 150 million kilometres away, are mind-bogglingly improbable. It's believed the chances of you and I existing are as inconceivable as 400 trillion/1 (that's a 4 with fourteen zeroes behind it) and I can't help but feel both incredibly special and insignificant at the same time.

You and I live in seemingly magical suits of meat and marrow, with around 30 trillion cells, 206 bones, 900 ligaments and 600 muscles. Your heart, your personal engine, beats around 100,000 times a day, pumping 7,600 litres of blood to ensure oxygen and carbon dioxide flow in and out of your system 24/7. Your lungs expand and contract around 22,000 times daily, non-stop for 4,000 weeks, the average life span of a human. *You are nothing short of a miracle*, and I truly believe that when we appreciate just how stupidly complex our bodies are, and how ridiculously incredible it is that we get to experience the world through them, those revelations might just act as a tiny catalyst to help us shift towards a perspective of appreciation and curiosity for what our body does for us – not just what it looks like. I hope this might inspire you to consider taking care of it that little bit more, with some of the information sprinkled throughout this book.

There's a lot of things in your body that are out of your control. For the most part it's just doing its thing on autopilot, with no say in the matter from you – whether it's your heart beating, your digestion digesting, your skin or hair growing, or any of the hundreds of thousands of metabolic processes happening at any given time just to keep your magical suit functioning.

But we're not powerlessly led by our bodies, far from it. We have an incredible amount of influence. Our heart rate can be changed through breath or movement, our digestion impacted through the food we eat, our overall wellbeing and recovery guided by how much we sleep we get, and of course, our mobility through the movement we expose our body to – these are all things we can influence. So while our DNA, the building blocks which make me and you, are sourced 50 per cent from your mum and 50 per cent from your dad, meaning that not only are you literally thrust into existence with zero say in who your parents are, but zero say in your unique genetic code, you still get to decide what you do with your body.

I like to imagine us as a ball of playdough. How big, what colour and how mouldable or stiff the playdough is, is predetermined and decided for us by what comes in our genetic box. But what we do with that playdough, what we decide to sculpt, is ultimately down to us and the decisions we make. In other words, you might not have chosen your body, but you are the guardian of it and you can get a hell of a lot out of it when you choose to focus on what you can control rather than what you can't.

I didn't write this book as the 'bible for your body', but rather a guide to get a little more out of it while it's here, so you can keep doing what you love, now and hopefully for a long time. You don't need to do everything in this book to build a body that lasts. Even the smallest changes can ripple and have a monumental impact down the line. But one thing I can say for certain is that you need to keep your body moving. While the moves in this book aren't *musts,* I really hope they've taught you something about you and your unique body and that you've gained a plethora of ideas for how to fit more movement into your life, now and for as long as possible.

No matter where you are right now, you have a choice to grab your bodily guardianship by the peanuts, marvel in the miracle that is your magical meat suit, the one true house you'll live in for the rest of your life, and choose to make it a nicer place to live by tending to your movement needs. Just don't forget to enjoy it while you have it, you only get one of them after all.

For the last time before I bid you farewell, I think it's time we took one more big deep BREATH together, and while we're at it, let's CHANGE PLACES too.

Best of luck on your body building mission, you little miracle.

All my love,

Adam xxx

Acknowledgements

I'd like to say a monumental thank you to the entire team at Century (Penguin Random House) for giving me the opportunity to put these words out into the world! Especially to Zennor Compton for being my number one advocate and encouraging me to step way out of my comfort zone to make this book happen. A special thank you to the wonderful Katherine Ormerod. This book wouldn't have been possible without you listening to and reading countless hours of ramblings and helping shape them into legitimate sentences. I'm incredibly thankful for your help and support, and to call you a friend.

Most importantly, thank you so much to you, for investing in me by buying this book. I can't begin to express how grateful I am that you're here, reading these words. I hope more than anything that you've gained something from reading this book, and that it will make your life that little bit better.

Thank you to my amazing parents for putting up with me for all these years and showing me what a loving family is made of. My brother Alec for literally saving my life and being my best friend. My sister Lucy for giving me a home while I worked out what the hell I wanted to do with my life. Most of all, thank you to my partner, Mar, my daughter Tara and my cat Gwen, for filling my life with so much love, purpose and zest: I love you.

Glossary

All the fancy fitness words demystified.

Abs the muscles across the front of your midriff. Made up of the rectus abdominus, transverse abdominus, external and internal oblique muscles. Otherwise known as the 'six pack'.

Abductors muscles responsible for moving your leg away from your body's midline.

Adductors muscles responsible for moving your leg towards your body's midline.

Anterior Pelvic Tilt a forward tilted pelvis, which is totally normal and seen in roughly 85 per cent of people.

Anteverted a body part that is sloping or tilting forward.

Biceps the muscle which lies on the front of the upper arm between the shoulder and the elbow, responsible for flexing your elbow. Aka your guns.

Cartilage strong connective tissue which protects your joints, reducing friction and rubbing. Think of it as a shock absorber throughout the body.

Circumduction circular movement from a ball and socket joint (the shoulder and hip). Think the action of circling your arms in a large gesture forward and backwards.

CNS central nervous system; the brain and the spinal cord.

Cold Flexibility movement without warming the body up. Muscles will be significantly tighter, and range of motion will be more limited.

Concentric Movement when a muscle shortens/contracts to make a movement. Think making your biceps bulge.

Deltoids a fancy word for shoulder muscles, which have three parts: front, middle and rear.

Dorsiflexion the act of lifting your foot up, towards your shin. Think the opposite of pointing your toes. Important for running, walking, balancing and squatting.

Eccentric Movement opposite of a concentric movement, when a muscle increases/relaxes to make a movement. Think lowering of a bicep curl.

Ehlers-Danlos Syndrome a group of rare inherited conditions that affect connective tissue creating very fragile joints.

Extension movement at a joint where the angle increased, such as straightening your leg.

External Rotation outwards rotation of the limbs away from the body. Think sitting cross-legged or losing an arm wrestle.

Flexion the opposite of extension. Movement at a joint where the angle decreases, such as bending your knee.

Goldilocks Zone not too little, not too much. The right amount of effort for you where we stress your body enough to cause adaption, but not so much that you cause overload and injury. This zone is unique to every person.

'Glutes' the muscles on your bum. Made up of the gluteus maximus (the main bit), gluteus medius (medium bit) and the gluteus minimus (the little bit). These muscles work to stabilise and move your hips in all kinds of ways.

Hamstrings or 'Hammys' muscles at the back of your thigh. Made up of three individual muscles: bicep femoris, semitendinosus, semimembranosus.

Hip Flexors five muscles in the front of the hip, responsible for flexing your hip. One of the muscles is actually a thigh muscle known as rectus femoris, while the other four are named the iliacus, psoas, pectineus and sartorius.

Hypermobility where joints can bend further than average.

Hypermobility affects between 10–25 per cent of the population and can lead to unstable joints and injury.

Internal Rotation inward rotation of the limbs towards the body. Think winning an arm wrestle.

Isometric a muscular contraction where the muscles don't change length. A static form of resistance training. Think about holding a plank.

Kyphosis an exaggerated, forward rounding of the upper back. The position that many of us sit in while working at a desk (*see* prawn).

Latissimus Dorsi or 'Lats' a broad, flat muscle on the back that covers most of your back, from your armpit down towards the bottom of your spine. Mainly responsible for adduction and extension of the arm at the shoulder.

Lateral Flexion bending a body part to the side. Think tilting your head sideways.

Ligaments bands of tough elastic tissue around the joints. Connect bone to bone, give your joints support and limit your movement.

Metabolites small molecules that supply our cells with energy, structural materials or enable the creation of other substances we need for growth, movement and survival.

Mobility movement ability

Obliques the muscles at the side of the abs. Essential for twisting.

Pavlov's Dogs an experiment to show how dogs could be conditioned to salivate at the sound of a bell (initially accompanied by a meal). The foundation of the ideas around classical behaviour conditioning.

'Pecs' pectoralis muscles connect the front of the chest to the upper arm.

Piriformis a flat, narrow muscle which runs from the lower spine through the bottom to the top of the thighs. Essential for nearly every movement in the lower body.

Plantar Fasciitis inflammation of a thick band of tissue that runs across the bottom of each foot and connects the heel bone to the toes. Can create chronic heel pain which in turn leads to foot, knee, hip or back problems.

Plantar Flexion pointing your toes away from the leg. Ballerina style.

Posterior Chain the back side of our body running from the back of your head to your heels. Kind of a big deal.

Prawn the shape many of us make with our spine while hunched over a computer. Beloved by the desk-dwelling diva (description very much my own).

Proprioception the sense that enables us to perceive the location, movement and action parts of the body including perception of joint position. Proprioception enables you to close your eyes and touch the end of your nose with your index finger perfectly. Proper superpower.

Pronated palm down grip, facing away from you; can also refer to joint tilt with pronated ankles meaning the foot rolls inwards and the arch flattens out.

Prone lying flat facing downwards.

Psoas a pair of large muscles which run from the spine to the groin on both sides of the body and work to flex the hips.

Quadratus Lumborum the deepest back muscle, often known as the 'QL'.

Quadriceps or 'Quads' the large muscle at the front of the thigh, responsible for extending the knee and flexing the hip. Made up of four muscles: rectus femoris, vastus lateralis, vastus intermedius, vastus medialis.

Range of Motion how far you can move or stretch a part of your body, such as a joint or a muscle.

'Rear Delts' posterior deltoids. The deltoids make up the rounded part of the shoulder and the back ones help you move your arm backwards.

Reciprocal Inhibition the relaxation of the muscles on one side of a joint to accommodate contraction on the other side.

Rep short for repetition, one single execution of an exercise, i.e. one push up.

Retroverted a body part that is sloping or tilting backwards.

Rhomboids two rhombus-shaped muscles associated with stability and movement of the shoulder girdle and blade (scapula).

Rotator Cuff Muscles group of four different muscles that help rotate and maintain stability within the shoulder: the supraspinatus, infraspinatus, subscapularis and teres minor.

RPE (Rate of Perceived Exertion) basically how hard you think you are pushing yourself, usually on a scale of 1–10. It's entirely subjective and is all about how the exercise is making you feel.

SAID Principle the theory that the human body adapts specifically to whatever demands we impose on it.

Scapula a fancy word for the shoulder blade. This blade of bone sits on the back of our ribcage and glides up, down and side to side as we move our shoulder.

Scoliosis where the spine twists and curves to the side.

Serratus Anterior a fan-shaped muscle which starts at the side of the chest below the armpit and connects to the scapula.

Shin Splints pain and tenderness along or just behind the large bone in the lower leg which often develops after intense exercise.

Soft Tissue ligaments, muscles and tendons. The soft areas of the body, which can become injured through sprains, strains or overload.

Spinal Erectors a set of muscles which straighten and rotate the back.

Supinated palm facing upwards. Can also refer to joint tilt with pronated ankles, meaning the foot rolls outwards and the arch curves.

Supine lying horizontally with the face upwards.

Suspension Trainer a system of ropes which allows you to use your own bodyweight to perform hundreds of exercises.

Tendons fibrous connective tissue that attaches your muscles to your bones.

Tennis Elbow inflammation of the tendons of the elbow caused by overuse of the muscles of the forearm.

Teres Major a small muscle that runs along the border of the shoulder blade. Helps with arm swinging and static posture.

Thoracic the middle section of the spine around the ribcage.

Trapezius Muscles or 'Traps' a large muscle that begins at the base of your skull and spans your entire upper back, across your shoulders and down to the middle of your spine in the shape of a kite. Divided into three sections: upper, middle and lower.

Triceps the large muscle on the underside of the upper arm.

Upper and Lower Cross Syndrome a theory that suggested weakness and tightness in either the upper or lower part of the body may cause pain and reduce range of motion, but is actually a load of nonsense.

Unilateral Training an exercise that only involves one limb like a single leg squat.

Vascularisation the process of growing blood vessels into a tissue to improve oxygen and nutrient supply. During exercise, the body needs more blood, which promotes the expansion of the blood vessel network, increasing blood flow and capillary density.

Vestibular System functions to detect the position and movement of our head in space, allowing for coordination of our eyes, posture and equilibrium. Found in the inner ear.

Warm Flexibility range of motion once your body has been warmed up and muscles loosened.

Winged Shoulder Blade also know as winged scapula or scapula alata. A sometimes-painful condition when the shoulder blade sticks out instead of lying close to the back of the ribcage.

Notes

WHAT IS MOBILITY?

1. Prathiyankara Shailendra, et al., 'Resistance training and mortality risk: A systematic review and meta-analysis', *American Journal of Preventive Medicine*, May 2022
2. Ewan Thomas et al., 'The relation between stretching typology and stretching duration: The effects on range of motion', *International Journal of Sports Medicine*, April 2018
3. Patroklos Androulakis-Korakakis, James P. Fisher and James Steele, 'The minimum effective training dose required to increase 1RM strength in resistance-trained men: A systematic review and meta-analysis', *Sports Medicine*, April 2020
4. Andrew Smythe, 'The straight and narrow of posture: Current clinical concepts', *Australian Journal of General Practice*, November 2021

WHAT DO YOU WANT?

1. Meningitis Research Foundation, www.meningitis.org

FLAMINGO DISCO: BALANCE

1. H. Tianwu et al., 'Effects of alcohol ingestion on vestibular function in postural control', *Acta Oto-Laryngologica*, 2009
2. H. Reimann et al., 'Interactions between different age-related factors affecting balance control in walking', *Frontiers in Sport and Active Living*, July 2020
3. World Health Organization, 'Falls', April 2021

NOTES

GET LOW: SQUAT

1. G. D'Onofrio et al., 'Musculoskeletal exercise: Its role in promoting health and longevity', *Progress in Cardiovascular Diseases*, March–April 2023
2. K. Sen and G. Prybutok, 'A quality mobility program reduces elderly social isolation', *Activities, Adaptation and Aging*, 2021
3. K. Edwards et al., 'Differences between race and sex in measures of hip morphology: A population-based comparative study', *Osteoarthritis and Cartilage*, February 2020
4. T. Yoshida et al., 'Change in Achilles tendon length after walking on treadmill with gradient', *Progress in Rehabilitation Medicine*, 2024

TOUCH YOUR TOOTSIES: FORWARD FOLD

1. E. B. Kroska, 'A meta-analysis of fear-avoidance and pain intensity: The paradox of chronic pain', *Scandinavian Journal of Pain*, October 2016

BOUNCE, BABY, BOUNCE: POGO

1. D. Manganaro et al., 'Anatomy, bony pelvis and lower limb, foot joints', StatPearls, August 2019
2. C. Agresta et al., 'Running injury paradigms and their influence on footwear design features and runner assessment methods: A focused review to advance evidence-based practice for running medicine clinicians', *Frontiers in Sport and Active Living*, March 2022

YOU SCRATCH YOUR BACK AND I'LL SCRATCH MINE: APLEY SCRATCH TEST

1. K. McQuade and G. Smidt, 'Dynamic scapulohumeral rhythm: The effects of external resistance during elevation of the arm in the scapular plane', *Journal of Orthopaedic & Sports Physical Therapy*, February 1998

PUSH IT REAL GOOD: THE PUSH UP

1. 'Falls', World Health Organization, April 2021
2. J. Yang et al., 'Association between push-up exercise capacity and future cardiovascular events among active adult men', *JAMA Network Open*, February 2019

LET'S HANG: DEAD HANG

1. R. Bohannon, 'Grip strength: An indispensable biomarker for older adults', *Clinical Interventions in Aging*, October 2019
2. Y. Wu et al., 'Association of grip strength with risk of all-cause mortality, cardiovascular diseases, and cancer in community-dwelling populations: A meta-analysis of prospective cohort studies', *Journal of the American Medical Directors Association*, June 2017
3. K. Forrest et al., 'Patterns and correlates of grip strength in older Americans', *Current Aging Science*, 2018

SIT DOWN, STAND UP: THE SIT AND RISE TEST

1. L. B. B. de Brito et al., 'Ability to sit and rise from the floor as a predictor of all-cause mortality', *European Journal of Preventive Cardiology*, 2014

MOVEMENT CHALLENGE SUMMARY

1. Javier Garcia-Campayo, Elena Asso and Marta Alda, 'Joint hypermobility and anxiety: The state of the art', *Current Psychiatry Reports*, 2011
2. Jane V. Simmonds and Rosemary J. Keer, 'Hypermobility and the hypermobility syndrome', *Manual Therapy*, November 2017
3. A. J. Haking and R. Grahame, 'A simple questionnaire to detect hypermobility: An adjunct to the Assessment of Patients with Diffuse Musculoskeletal Pain', *International Journal of Clinical Practice*, April 2003

PERFECT POSTURE

1. Sai Kripa and Harmanpreet Kaur, 'Identifying relations between posture and pain in lower back pain patients: A narrative review', *Bulletin of Faculty of Physical Therapy*, December 2021

2. J. Hartvigsen et al., 'What low back pain is and why we need to pay attention', *Lancet Oncology*, 2018

3. 'Global, regional, and national burden of low back pain, 1990–2020, its attributable risk factors, and projections to 2050: A systematic analysis of the global burden of disease study 2021', *The Lancet Rheumatology*, June 2023

4. J. D. Cassidy, L. J. Carroll and P. Côté, 'The Saskatchewan health and back pain survey. The prevalence of low back pain and related disability in Saskatchewan adults', *Spine*, September 1998

5. Tarcisio F. de Campos et al., 'Prognosis of a new episode of low-back pain in a community inception cohort', *European Journal of Pain*, 2023

6. R. A. Laird, J. Gilbert, P. Kent et al., 'Comparing lumbo-pelvic kinematics in people with and without back pain: A systematic review and meta-analysis', *BMC Musculoskeletal Disorders*, 2014

7. Sanne Toftgaard Christensen, Jan Hartvigsen, 'Spinal curves and health: A systematic critical review of the epidemiological literature dealing with associations between sagittal spinal curves and health', *Journal of Manipulative and Physiological Therapeutics*, 2008

8. K. V. Richards et al., 'Is neck posture subgroup in late adolescence a risk factor for persistent neck pain in young adults? A prospective study', *Physical Therapy and Rehabilitation Journal*, March 2021

9. Diane Slater et al., '"Sit Up Straight": Time to re-evaluate', *The Journal of Orthopaedic and Sports Physical Therapy*, August 2019

BUILDING THE HABIT

1. B. J. Schoenfeld et al., 'Inter-set stretch: A potential time-efficient strategy for enhancing skeletal muscle adaptations', *Frontiers in Sports and Active Living*, November 2022

MOVING MORE THROUGHOUT THE DAY

1. A. Carron et al., 'Social influence and exercise: A meta-analysis, *Journal of Sport and Exercise Psychology*, 1996
2. S. Burke et al., 'Group versus individual approach? A meta-analysis of the effectiveness of interventions to promote physical activity', *International Review of Sport and Exercise Psychology*, November 2005
3. Jordan D. Miller et al., 'Skeletal muscle pump versus respiratory muscle pump: modulation of venous return from the locomotor limb in humans', *The Journal of Physiology*, March 2005
4. Paul Kelly, Chloë Williamson, Alisa G. Niven et al., 'Walking on sunshine: Scoping review of the evidence for walking and mental health', *British Journal of Sports Medicine*, May 2018
5. Maciej Banach et al., 'The association between daily step count and all-cause and cardiovascular mortality: A meta-analysis', *European Journal of Preventive Cardiology*, December 2023
6. Julia Lynch et al., 'Classroom movement breaks and physically active learning are feasible, reduce sedentary behaviour and fatigue and may increase focus in university students: A systemic review and meta-analysis', *International Journal of Environmental Research and Public Health*, June 2022
7. A. J. Daly-Smith et al., 'Systematic review of acute physically active learning and classroom movement breaks on children's physical activity, cognition, academic performance and classroom behaviour: Understanding critical design features', *BMJ Open Sport and Exercise Medicine*, March 2018

INJURY PREVENTION

1. A. J. Fradkin et al., 'Effects of warming-up on physical performance: A systematic review with meta-analysis', *Journal of Strength and Conditioning Research*, January 2010
2. P. Bishop et al., 'Warm-up and stretching in the prevention of muscular injury', *Sports Medicine*, October 2007
3. A. J. Fradkin et al., 'Does warming up prevent injury in sport?: The evidence from randomised controlled trials?', *Journal of Science and Medicine in Sport*, June 2006

4. P. Bishop et al., 'Warm-up and stretching in the prevention of muscular injury', *Sports Medicine*, October 2007

INJURY, RECOVERY AND WORKING AROUND PAIN

1. Dr G. Mirkin, 'Why Ice Delays Recovery', https://drmirkin.com/fitness/why-ice-delays-recovery.html, September 2015
2. B. Dubois and J. F. Esculier, 'Soft-tissue injuries simply need PEACE and LOVE', *British Journal of Sports Medicine*, August 2019
3. A. Hendy et al., 'Cross education and immobilisation: Mechanisms and implications for injury rehabilitation', *Journal of Science and Medicine in Sport*, March 2012
4. G. Lehman, 'Do Our Patients Need Fixing? Or Do They Need a Bigger Cup?', *Reconciling Biomechanics with Pain Science*, May 2018

THE BIG PICTURE

1. G. Belenky et al., 'Patterns of performance degradation and restoration during sleep restriction and subsequent recovery: A sleep dose-response study', *Journal of Sleep Research*, March 2003
2. Yuri Milaneschi et al., 'Mediterranean diet and mobility decline in older persons', *Experimental Gerontology*, April 2011

HIDDEN BENEFITS OF MOBILITY TRAINING

1. M. Pearce et al., 'Association between physical activity and risk of depression: A systematic review and meta-analysis', *JAMA Psychiatry*, June 2022

Index

Page references in *italics* indicate images.